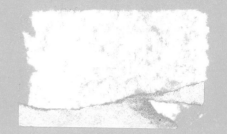

Leg and Foot Ulcers

Leg and Foot Ulcers
A Clinician's Guide

Vincent Falanga
MD, FACP
Associate Professor of Dermatology and Medicine

William H. Eaglstein
MD
Chairman and Harvey Blank Professor

Department of Dermatology and Cutaneous Surgery
University of Miami School of Medicine
Miami, Florida, USA

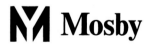 Mosby

St. Louis   Baltimore   Boston   Carlsbad   Chicago   Naples   New York   Philadelphia   Portland
London   Madrid   Mexico City   Singapore   Sydney   Tokyo   Toronto   Wiesbaden

Martin Dunitz

© Martin Dunitz Limited 1995

First published in the United Kingdom in 1995
by Martin Dunitz Ltd, The Livery House, 7–9 Pratt Street, London NW1 0AE

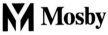 **Mosby**
Dedicated to Publishing Excellence
**A Times Mirror
Company**

Distributed in the U.S.A. and Canada by
Mosby–Year Book
11830 Westline Industrial Drive
St. Louis, Missouri 63146

Library of Congress Cataloguing-in-Publication Data applied for

ISBN 1 85317 173 5

Printed and bound in Singapore

Contents

Dedicated to the memory of our fathers

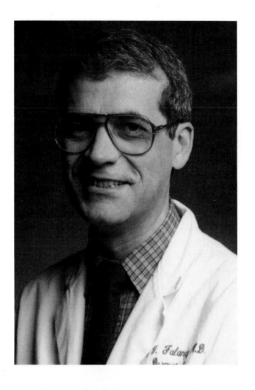

Dr Falanga is currently an Associate Professor of Medicine and Dermatology at the University of Miami School of Medicine. A diplomate of the American Boards of Internal Medicine and Dermatology, Dr Falanga is a fellow of the American College of Physicians and a member of the Wound Healing Society, the American College of Rheumatology, the American Academy of Dermatology and the Society of Investigative Dermatology. He is on the Editorial Board of the *Journal of Dermatologic Surgery and Oncology* and the *Journal of the European Academy of Dermatology and Venereology*, and serves as an associate editor for *Wounds*. He is a consultant to the National Institutes of Health and is active in drug research and development, particularly with regard to the treatment of chronic wounds. The author of more than 170 publications, most of them related to wound repair and fibrosis, Dr Falanga is a graduate of Harvard Medical School. His internship and residency in medicine were at the University of Miami and were followed by a dermatology residency at the University of Pennsylvania. In addition to his interest in the basic research aspects of wound healing and fibrosis, Dr Falanga is actively involved in the care of patients with chronic wounds and in testing new therapies for accelerating wound repair. Since 1986, he has directed a wound healing fellowship program at the University of Miami.

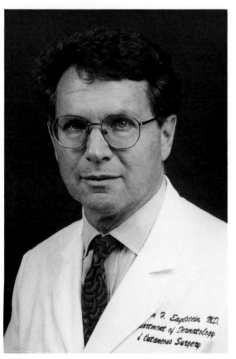

Currently the Harvey Blank Professor and Chairman of the Department of Dermatology and Cutaneous Surgery at the University of Miami School of Medicine, Dr Eaglstein was previously Chairman of the Department of Dermatology, University of Pittsburgh, from 1980 to 1986. He is a member of the Board of Directors of the Society of Investigative Dermatology, the Wound Healing Society and the Association of Professors of Dermatology, as well as a consultant to the Food and Drug Administration. He has also served on the Board of Directors of the American Academy of Dermatology, and in 1986–7 was a Robert Wood Johnson Health Policy Fellow. In 1993 he was appointed to the US Department of Health and Human Services' National Advisory Board for Arthritis and Musculoskeletal and Skin Diseases. The author of more than 140 publications, Dr Eaglstein is a native of Kansas City, Missouri, and a graduate of the University of Missouri School of Medicine. In addition to his interest in wound repair and the etiology of chronic wounds, he is active in drug development and regulatory affairs.

Acknowledgments

The publishers are grateful to the following for permission to reproduce copyright illustrations:

American Medical Association — Figure 13.16a from *Arch Dermatol* (1986) **122**: Falanga V, Fine MJ, Kapoor WN, The cutaneous manifestations of cholesterol crystal embolization, 1194–1198

Elsevier Science Inc. — Figures 12.8, 13.6, 13.10a, 13.10b, 14.12, 16.7a, 16.7b, 16.7c from *J Dermatol Surg Oncol* (1992) **18**: Falanga V, Kirsner RS, Katz MM, et al, Pericapillary fibrin cuffs in venous ulceration, 409–414; (1993) **19**: Harris B, Eaglstein WH, Falanga V, Basal cell carcinoma arising in venous ulcers and mimicking granulation tissue, 150–152; Falanga V, Venous ulceration, 764–771

Mosby–Year Book, Inc. — Figure 6.9 from *J Am Acad Dermatol* (1993) **28**: Kirsner RS, Pardes JB, Eaglstein WH, et al, The clinical spectrum of lipodermatosclerosis, 623–627

Introduction

For the last 10 years we have jointly sponsored a leg ulcer program. The principal elements of this program are a weekly outpatient session, a training program for wound healing fellows, inpatient care of leg ulcers, a program of controlled therapeutic trials, and a series of studies aimed at understanding the etiology and pathophysiology of venous ulceration.

This book comes primarily from the authors' shared experience in the leg ulcer program, especially in outpatients. Our interest in leg and foot ulcers had several roots. First, our experience with occlusive dressings in experimental animals led to a desire to apply occlusive dressings to leg ulcers. Secondly, publication by British surgeons Browse and Burnand of the pericapillary fibrin hypothesis of venous leg ulcer pathogenesis made us interested in caring for leg ulcers. Their hypothesis suggested that leg ulcer problems might be approached on a rational, rather than empiric, basis. One of us (VF) had an antecedent interest in systemic sclerosis and other rheumatologic conditions in which there is a high incidence of chronic wounds including leg and foot ulcers. The other (WHE) had an antecedent interest in wound healing which seemed linked at least intellectually to non-healing.

We hope this book distills into a modest number of pictures and words much of the clinical information we have learned about leg and foot ulcers over the past decade. It is designed to be used in the office where patients' ulcers can be compared to the photographs and situations, and at home, where the book can be read as a series of semi-independent vignettes. It is not written for the beginning doctor, but should be very helpful for the doctor beginning to care for leg and foot ulcers. It is not a comprehensive textbook about leg and foot ulcers but rather is intended to show an array of clinical appearances.

The captions contain information or thinking that has helped us in planning patient management. We have not described all the findings in each photograph. We have, however, tried to relate the information and thoughts about each situation which we have found useful for making a diagnosis and giving treatments. Toward that end, the book is laid out according to clinical issue, which allows the figures, each showing a clinical situation, to be grouped in a clinically relevant manner. Situations in which factors away from the ulcer area guide thinking and therapy are in one section; situations in which the appearance of the ulcer bed guide the physician is in another, and so forth. The higher number of illustrations in some categories is generally the result of how useful those observations have been to us in both diagnosis and treatment. Rarely, a figure is shown more than once to make different points. Although each section can stand on its own, we have resisted the common practice to artificially group all similar clinical problems together within each section. A brief glossary of selected terms is included to avoid repeating definitions and details of pathophysiologic points and treatment modalities that are mentioned more frequently. The bibliography consists of background or original articles for the ideas expressed in this work. We have included articles that may express a different point of view. There has been a great deal of interest in leg ulcers over the last decade, and we have obviously not been able to include all worthy publications pertinent to our work.

Finally, we are all too aware of the anecdotal or scientifically unproven nature of many points made in this book. We offer them as "working facts" until studies and better observations appear. Our aim is to assist those who, as us, need to care for the leg ulcer patients today.

Shortly after starting to treat leg and foot ulcers, we realized that they are not the domain or category of any one specialty. People trained in vascular surgery, dermatology, rheumatology, diabetology, family and general medicine, podiatry, and nursing all care for leg and foot ulcers. There is not a clear cut body of literature on the subject or a journal dealing specifically with leg ulcers. We also quickly realized that, as compared to Europeans, Americans have been generally uninterested in leg ulcers. We think that American physicians recently have become more interested, and we hope that this book will stimulate American doctors, students, and nurses to develop the habit we observed among Japanese dermatology students of frequently comparing photographs in picture books and atlases with clinical problems observed in their patients. Such direct visual comparing may be more natural to people whose language is pictographic rather than alphabetic. We urge those who use this book to look through the photographs after they see their patients. We hope they will find a look-alike situation and use the information.

Finally, we want to acknowledge and thank the many colleagues, associates, and employees whose assistance made this book possible. Special thanks go to our wound healing fellows who have assisted us in caring for patients with leg and foot ulcers: Brian Bucalo, Adam Greenberg, Brian Harris, Todd Helfman, Matthew Katz, Robert Kirsner, Albert Nemeth and Jeffrey Pardes. We gratefully acknowledge the help of Ms Lisa Peerson and Ms Polly Carson, who have been instrumental in the care of many of the patients presented in this book. We also wish to thank Ms Cari Martinez for her secretarial work.

I   AWAY FROM THE ULCER AREA

Introduction

In the evaluation of patients with ulcers, we have found it necessary to resist the temptation to focus immediately on the ulcer itself. Signs and symptoms which are somewhat distant from the ulcer may be helpful in making or excluding a diagnosis. Knowledge of the past medical history and careful physical examination are essential. Thus, ulcers associated with or caused by connective tissue diseases, especially rheumatoid arthritis, arterial insufficiency and neuropathy are most likely to be understood as a result of findings away from the ulcer itself. Rheumatoid arthritis, vasculitis, systemic sclerosis, and periarteritis nodosa are among the connective tissue diseases with which leg ulcers occur. In time, the experienced clinician will look for specific signs and information. The presence of sclerodactyly will suggest systemic sclerosis. The joint disfigurement of rheumatoid arthritis in a patient with a typical ulceration strongly suggests the diagnosis of pyoderma gangrenosum. The sternal scar from coronary bypass surgery suggests concomitant arterial insufficiency. The cushingoid appearance of a patient will tell us that the inflammation necessary for proper wound healing may be absent or inadequate because of the use of corticosteroids. Similarly, the presence of arthritis indicates a high likelihood that the patient is taking large doses of aspirin and non-steroidal inflammatory drugs, which may impair the healing process.

Management, too, will be affected by the underlying systemic disease. For example, healing in patients who are on systemic corticosteroids can be achieved by the application of retinoic acid to the wound bed. With regard to arterial insufficiency, it is worth remembering that distal pulses may be present even in arterial disease and that arterial ulcers are often surrounded by a paradoxical increased erythema. This erythema is due to maximal vasodilatation and may be falsely viewed as a sign of adequate circulation and delay appropriate treatment. A history of diabetes mellitus will lead us to perform a neurological exam to exclude peripheral neuropathy. The presence of a neuropathy will in turn focus our attention on the patient's weight bearing and to pressure points in his shoes. In this section, we have outlined many of these situations. Overall, our advice is to always "step back" and regard the patient as a whole before focusing on the ulceration that brought him to our office.

1 Connective tissue diseases

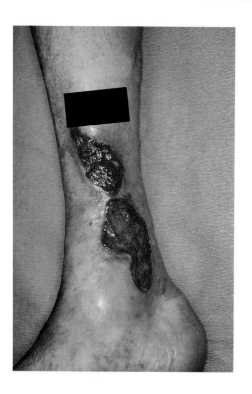

Figure 1.1
Rheumatoid ulceration

This 58-year-old woman with rheumatoid arthritis has longstanding leg ulcerations. She had no laboratory evidence of venous or arterial disease. A biopsy from the edge of one of the ulcerations did not show vasculitis. This smooth, undulating, "geographic" shape is typical of rheumatoid ulcers and is not usually found with venous ulcers. She did not have leukopenia, as one would find with Felty's syndrome.

Figure 1.2
Connective tissue disease and ulcer

This circumferential ulceration has never been satisfactorily classified. The patient has Raynaud's disease and arthritis and has had this ulceration for over 12 years. Venous and arterial studies are normal. A biopsy from the ulcer's edge did not show pericapillary fibrin, a finding that strongly argues against a venous etiology. Hydrocolloid dressing therapy was given to stimulate the formation of granulation tissue. The dressing was removed moments before this photograph was made. Some of the ulcer edges are hydrated and white from the use of occlusion therapy. Note the early buds of granulation tissue within the center portion of the ulcer bed.

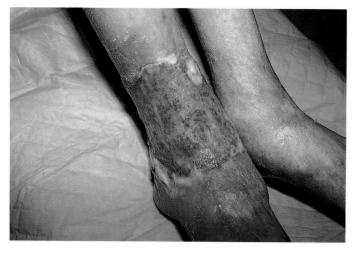

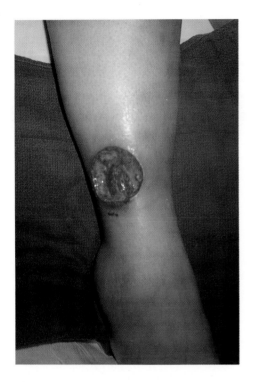

Figure 1.3
Ulcer in a woman with systemic lupus erythematosus

This ulcer developed while the patient was taking oral corticosteroids for systemic complications of her disease. Many biopsies failed to show vasculitis. Treatment with topically applied retinoic acid produced a mild improvement in the granulation tissue but was inadequate. She was successfully treated by split-thickness grafting. Grafting of ulcers due to chronic inflammatory conditions is often successful.

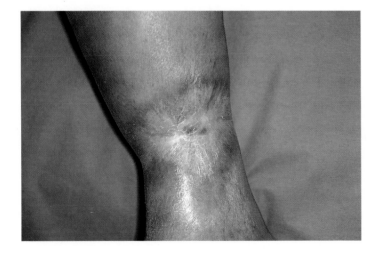

Figure 1.4
Pyoderma gangrenosum and rheumatoid arthritis

This woman healed with systemic corticosteroid treatment. The amount of scarring shown in this illustration is not unusual.

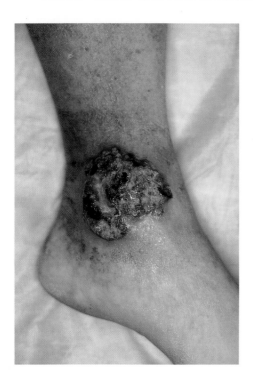

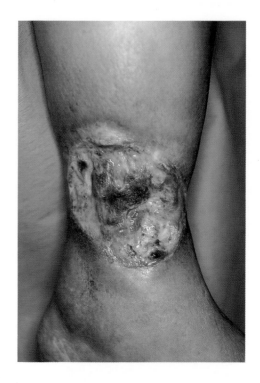

Figure 1.5
Pyoderma gangrenosum in the venous ulcer area

Although the location was typical for a venous ulcer, the scalloped edges suggested pyoderma gangrenosum. This patient healed with systemic corticosteroid therapy.

Figure 1.6
Rheumatoid arthritis and pyoderma gangrenosum

This is a well known association. As in this particular patient, pyoderma gangrenosum does not always have the typical clear ulcer bed often described.

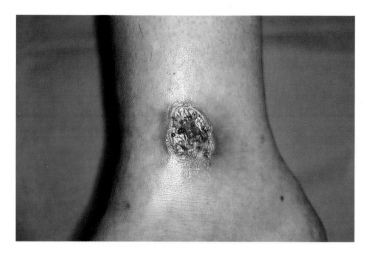

Figure 1.7a
Antiphospholipid syndrome

This woman with systemic lupus erythematosus had the antiphospholipid syndrome. In addition to the leg ulcer, she had a history of recurrent abortions. Stanozolol was used in the hope that the fibrinolytic activity of this androgen would lyse the intravascular fibrin thrombi of this condition. Her pain resolved and the ulcer improved considerably but did not heal completely with stanozolol therapy.

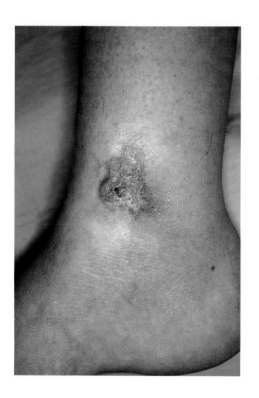

Figure 1.7b
Antiphospholipid syndrome — healed ulcer

In the same patient, a single treatment with intralesional triamcinolone acetonide (5 mg/ml) finally produced total closure and the ulcer has not recurred in nine months.

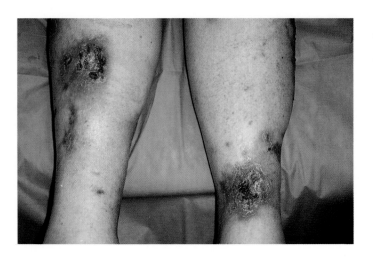

Figure 1.8a
Pyoderma gangrenosum

This man had diabetes but no risk factors for pyoderma gangrenosum. Wound cultures were negative for pathogens, and he responded to i.v. pulse corticosteroid therapy. The lesion with the punched-out areas of ulceration is characteristic.

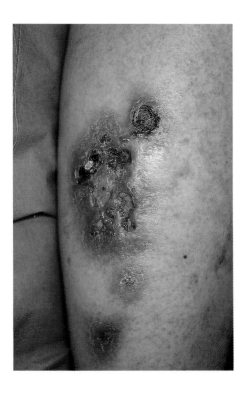

Figure 1.8b
Pyoderma gangrenosum/Close-up

The mixture of healed sites and draining sinuses in red, indurated and boggy parts of the lesion is common in lesions of pyoderma gangrenosum.

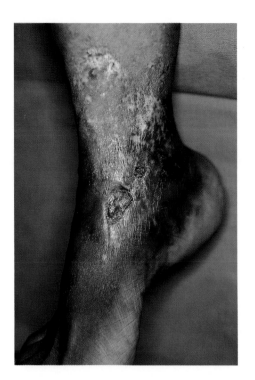

Figure 1.9
Very painful ulcer in a patient with systemic lupus erythematosus

This middle aged woman with systemic lupus erythematosus had the clinical picture of atrophie blanche. The episodic ulcerations were extremely painful. Biopsies did not show intravascular fibrin thrombi; rather, the histology was consistent with venous ulceration. Cryofibrinogen, anti-cardiolipin antibodies and cryoglobulin studies on this patient were normal. Because of the extreme pain caused by her ulcer she was treated with stanozolol. The response was prompt and impressive with complete pain relief within a few days. She is one of several people with painful ulcerations that could not be attributed to cryofibrinogenemia, cryoglobulinemia, or the antiphospholipid syndrome but which have responded to stanozolol.

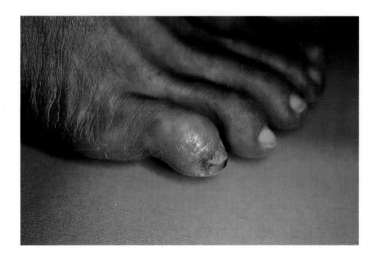

Figure 1.10
Persistent toe infection

This woman with systemic sclerosis had pain, tenderness and drainage from the fifth toe for several months. There was no evidence of osteomyelitis. The infection cleared up only after continuing systemic antibiotics for over two months. In our experience, infected fibrotic skin is usually slow in its response to antibiotics, perhaps as a result of impaired blood flow.

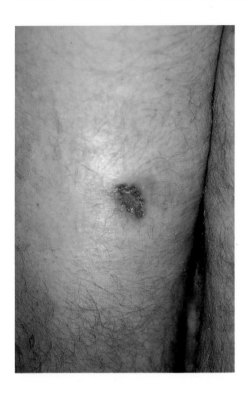

Figure 1.11a
Pyoderma gangrenosum

The edges of this ulcer are highly suggestive of this condition. There were similar ulcers on many parts of this patient's body.

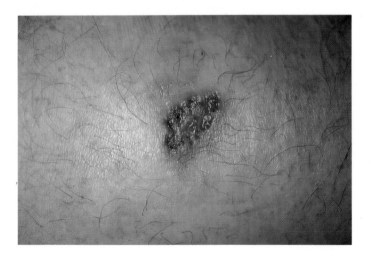

Figure 1.11b
Pyoderma gangrenosum/Follow up

The patient responded promptly to pulse corticosteroid therapy (approximately 1 g of solumedrol i.v. daily for 3–5 days) and was maintained free of lesions with clofazamine 200 mg twice daily.

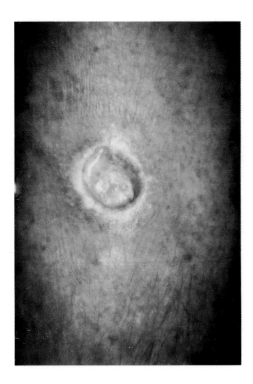

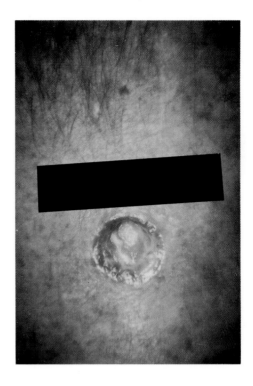

Figure 1.12a
Ulceration in an immunocompromised patient: treatment with retinoic acid

This 62-year-old man was being treated with prednisone because of temporal arteritis. He developed an ulceration on his shin after a fall, and the ulcer did not show any evidence of reepithelialization for five months. The ulcer has only pale granulation tissue. These are characteristic findings in non-healing ulcerations in immunocompromised patients.

Figure 1.12b
Ulceration in an immunocompromised patient: treatment with retinoic acid/Follow up

Treatment was initiated with nightly application of 0.05% retinoic acid cream applied to the base of the ulceration after protection of the surrounding skin with petrolatum. Vitamin A and derivatives have been shown to offset the deleterious effects of prednisone on healing. With only one week of retinoic acid, increased and redder granulation tissue is seen at the edges of the ulceration.

Continued

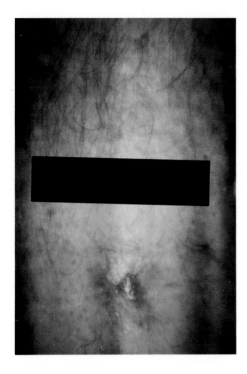

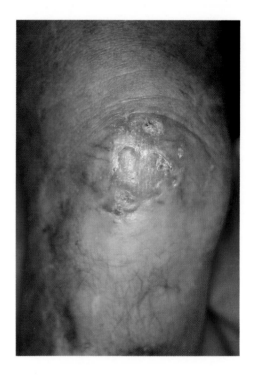

Figure 1.12c
Ulceration in an immunocompromised patient: treatment with retinoic acid/Follow up

After approximately four months of treatment, the ulcer is filled with good granulation tissue and is smaller. The ulcer went on to heal after an additional two months of retinoic acid. The prednisone for this patient's temporal arteritis was maintained at a dosage of 10 mg/day throughout treatment with retinoic acid.

Figure 1.13
Calcinosis

The entire leg in this patient with CREST syndrome was affected by calcinosis. As observed in this photograph, these areas often became ulcerated and would not heal.

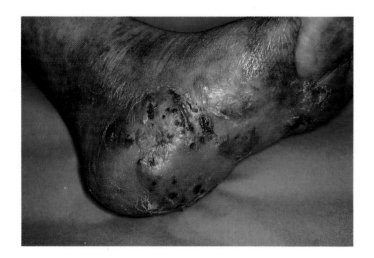

Figure 1.14a
Granulomatous pyoderma gangrenosum

This rare variant of pyoderma gangrenosum is not well recognized. In this patient the lesion is mycetoma-like and covers most of the sole of the foot. Many cultures of biopsy material as well as special histologic stains failed to detect fungi or mycobacteria. This painful, incapacitating, and growing lesion finally responded to pulse corticosteroid therapy.

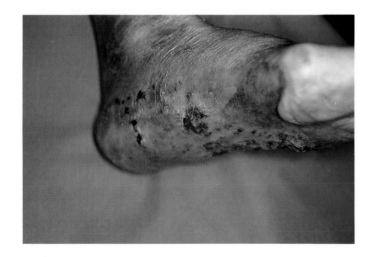

Figure 1.14b
Granulomatous pyoderma gangrenosum/Follow-up

One week after steroid pulse therapy the swelling and tissue infiltration have resolved dramatically. Now the sites of grafts placed earlier in the course of unsuccessful therapies can be seen proximal to the metatarsal area. The superficial crusting and ulceration resolved within two weeks.

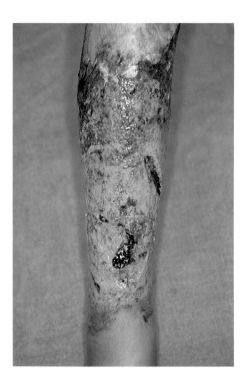

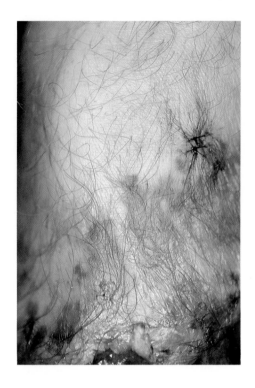

Figure 1.15a
Vasculitis

For many years this man had recurrent episodes of an eruption on his lower extremities that left ashy hyperpigmented lesions. The current and more severe episode resulted in total denudation with areas of deeper necrosis. The elliptical wound on the right side of this picture is the site of a large inconclusive surgical biopsy. The pain was excruciating, and he had already been hospitalized elsewhere without improvement after several courses of intravenous antibiotics.

Figure 1.15b
Vasculitis/Close-up

The clue to diagnosis is at the superior edge of this markedly tender widespread ulcerative condition. The purple-red, hemorrhagic and blistering edge suggests a vasculitis. The biopsy of this edge showed leukocytoclastic vasculitis. The patient responded dramatically to treatment with systemic corticosteroids.

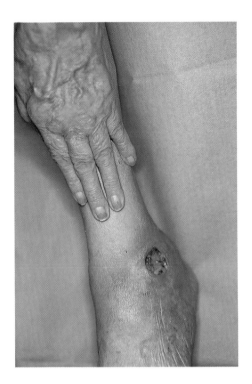

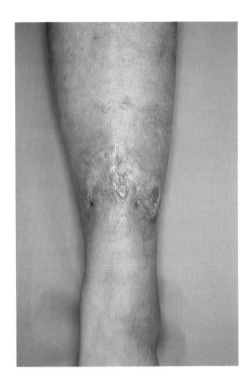

Figure 1.16
Ulcer in a patient with rheumatoid arthritis

Many patients with ulcers have extremely complicated histories and a variety of diseases which might account for, or contribute to, their ulcers. This woman had rheumatoid arthritis, a history of pyoderma gangrenosum, and severe arterial insufficiency. She did not respond to hyperbaric oxygen treatment but did improve somewhat with intravenous pulse corticosteroid therapy.

Figure 1.17
Unusual ulceration in a diabetic patient

The appearance of this ulcer in a female diabetic patient suggested either pyoderma gangrenosum or necrobiosis lipoidica diabeticorum. A biopsy showed no evidence of the latter. The ulcer began to heal with intralesional injections of corticosteroids. We believe she had pyoderma gangrenosum.

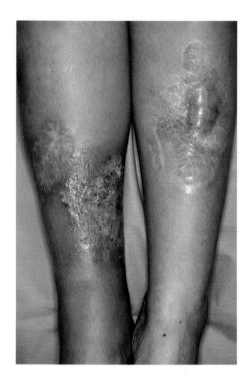

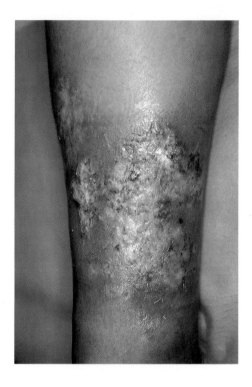

Figure 1.18a
Pyoderma gangrenosum

This female patient shows a good example of severe scarring produced by pyoderma gang-renosum.

Figure 1.18b
Pyoderma gangrenosum/Close-up

Her new ulcers healed with 60 mg/day of oral prednisone. High doses (60 mg of prednisone or higher) of corticosteroids are often necessary. Intralesional steroids have also been effective.

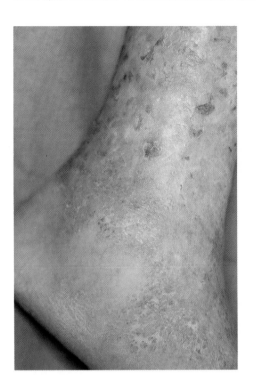

Figure 1.19a
Atrophie blanche and recurrent ulcerations

The non-specific nature of atrophie blanche is illustrated in this patient. Atrophie blanche is not a specific clinical entity but occurs in the setting of various etiologies, including venous and arterial disease, vasculitis, cryofibrinogenemia and cryoglobulinemia.

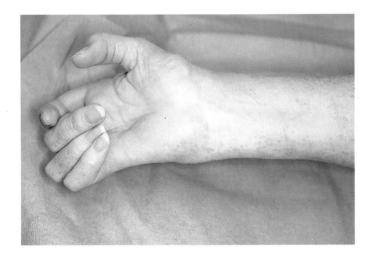

Figure 1.19b
Atrophie blanche and recurrent ulcerations/Arm lesions

In addition, the patient had a red papular eruption of the forearm and hand which showed granulomas histologically. Both her children have rheumatoid arthritis and similar papular eruptions.

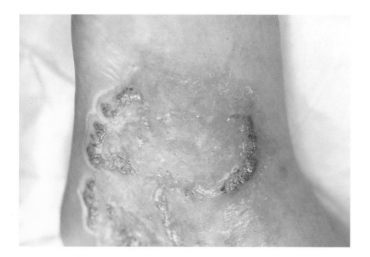

Figure 1.20
Pyoderma gangrenosum

The rolled scalloped edges are suggestive of pyoderma gangrenosum. Intralesional steroid treatments had induced a remission. Now, the process is "breaking through".

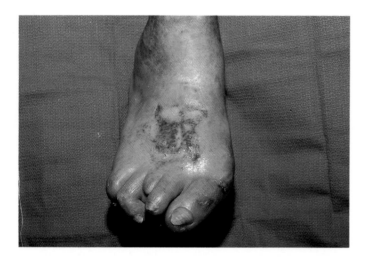

Figure 1.21
Rheumatoid ulcer

This female patient has rheumatoid arthritis and recurrent ulcers in unusual locations with unusual shapes.

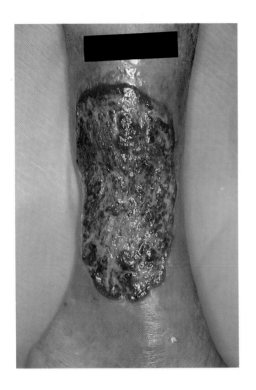

Figure 1.22
Rheumatoid ulcer

This large clean looking ulcer is surrounded by soft, normal appearing tissue. Biopsies from the ulcer's edge as well as vascular studies did not produce any evidence of venous or arterial disease. The patient has had rheumatoid arthritis for many years.

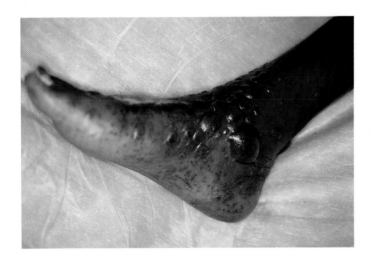

Figure 1.23
Leukocytoclastic vasculitis with blister

Biopsy of this acute blistering eruption showed leukocytoclastic vasculitis. The ulcers resulting from this will heal within a few weeks.

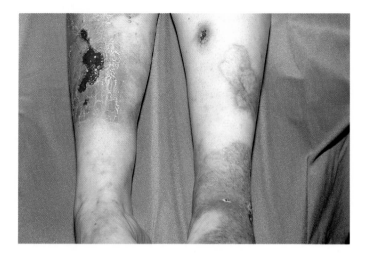

Figure 1.24
Pyoderma gangrenosum and Behçet's disease

The hyperpigmented rim of healed lesions is suggestive. The ulcer healed after intravenous pulse corticosteroids and oral azathioprine.

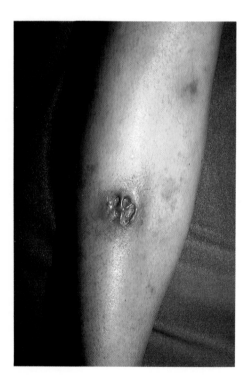

Figure 1.25
Pyoderma gangrenosum

The fenestrations are highly suggestive. The non-ulcerated, red, indurated, "satellite" lesion in the superior portion of this patient's leg seems ready to ulcerate.

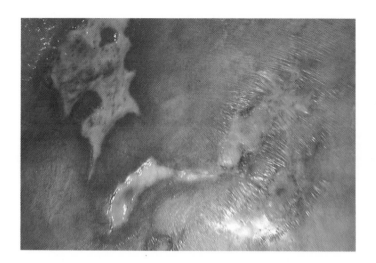

Figure 1.26
"Angular" ulcers

This 56-year-old woman with CREST developed these non-healing ulcers in many areas of her body, including her legs. The unusual irregular and "angular" appearance may at first suggest factitial disease. The histology was non-specific. We have seen similar ulcers in patients with dermatomyositis.

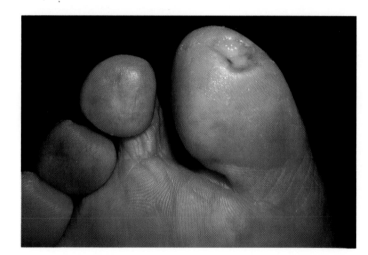

Figure 1.27
Toe ulcer in systemic sclerosis

Raynaud's phenomenon in these patients is due in large part to intimal proliferation and a fixed vascular defect. For this reason, Raynaud's phenomenon in systemic sclerosis does not respond as well to vasodilators as Raynaud's phenomenon associated with other connective tissue disease, in which spasm is the predominant factor. Digital ulcers in these patients do not reepithelialize readily. However, the formation of granulation tissue can often be stimulated by occlusive dressings.

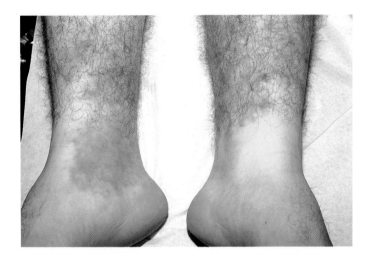

Figure 1.28a
Cutaneous periarteritis nodosa

This 19-year-old man had a persistent rash and periodic ulcerations since childhood. The left ankle hyperpigmentation is a clue to previous episodes of his condition. An excisional biopsy of an acute lesion on his leg showed a intense inflammatory process destroying a medium-sized blood vessel in the subcutaneous tissue. He had no systemic complications.

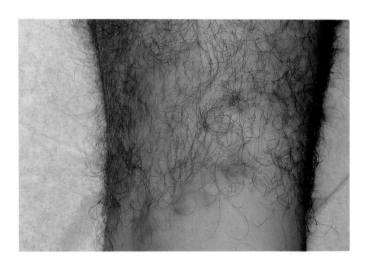

Figure 1.28b
Cutaneous periarteritis nodosa/ Close-up

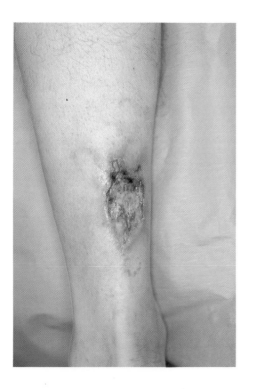

Figure 1.29
Cryofibrinogenemia

This painful non-healing ulcer in a middle aged woman with systemic lupus erythematosus was due to cryofibrinogenemia. She had detectable plasma levels of cryofibrinogen, and intravascular fibrin thrombi were present histologically. The area to be biopsied is marked in ink at the superior border of the ulcer. The ulcer healed with stanozolol therapy.

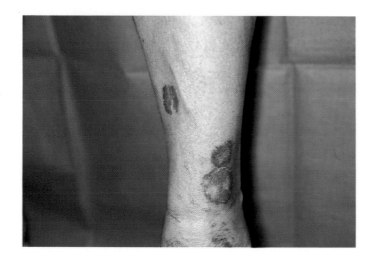

Figure 1.30
Subacute lupus erythematosus

These annular lesions, which would often develop erosions, were also present on this female patient's arms and trunk. The lesions improved markedly with hydroxychloroquine sulfate (Plaquenyl).

2 Diminished or absent pulses

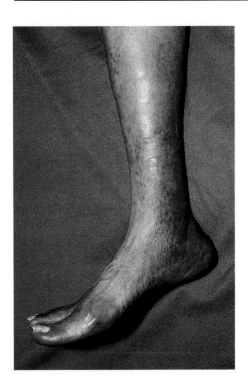

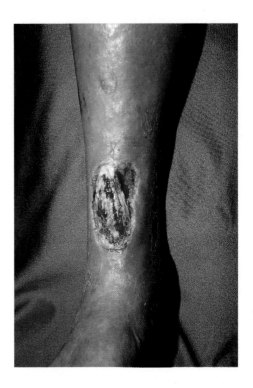

Figure 2.1
Combined arterial and venous insufficiency

This 70-year-old woman had many varicosities extending from the foot to the upper portion of her leg. In a dependent position her toes were purple-red. There was also evidence of onychomycosis. Her skin was shiny and hairless, and was cool to touch, especially on the foot. No pedal pulses were detectable. This is an example of combined venous and arterial insufficiency, a combination reported to occur in up to 20% of elderly patients with venous disease.

Figure 2.2
Inoperable arterial disease with ulceration and exposed tendon

In similar cases, some have advocated scoring the tendon with a scalpel to stimulate granulation tissue growth. This approach was not successful for this patient.

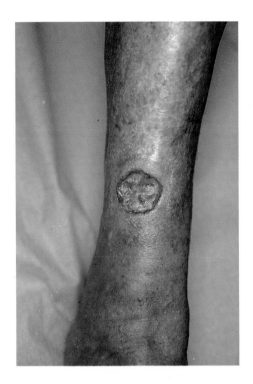

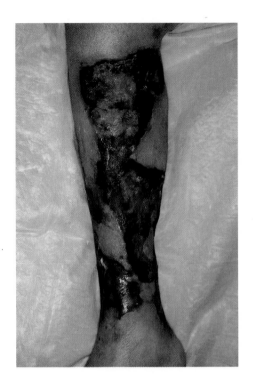

Figure 2.3
Punched-out ulcer

This woman has a history of recurrent lesions which have been labeled pyoderma gangrenosum. Studies showed arterial insufficiency. A punched-out ulcer may be due to arterial insufficiency or inflammatory conditions.

Figure 2.4
Sudden widespread necrosis and ulceration

This woman in her 70s developed these necrotic ulcerations quite suddenly, together with acute renal failure. The diagnosis of periarteritis nodosa was considered but arteriography showed severe atherosclerotic vascular disease. No evidence of sepsis was found.

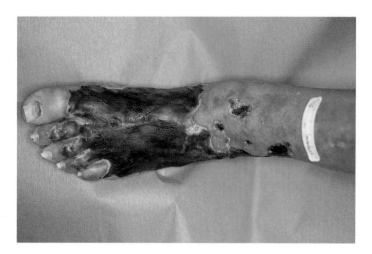

Figure 2.5a
Massive necrosis following cardiac resuscitation

This man with advanced coronary artery disease had a cardiac arrest in the hospital and was resuscitated within minutes. Two days later this extensive necrosis of his feet became evident.

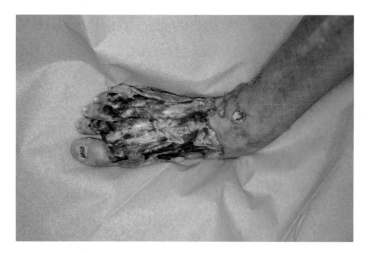

Figure 2.5b
Massive necrosis following cardiac resuscitation/Follow up

The patient's other foot, days later. *Pseudomonas aeruginosa* grew from these necrotic ulcers. He kept refusing amputation and died of Pseudomonas septicemia several weeks later.

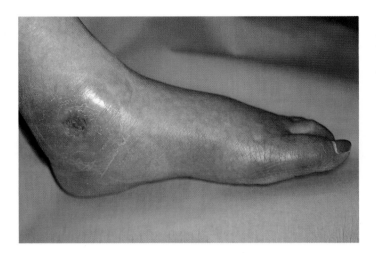

Figure 2.6
Multiple sclerosis with purple foot

Judging from the color of the foot and diminished pedal pulses, we felt certain this female patient had severe arterial insufficiency. However, this was not confirmed by arteriography. We have not had the opportunity to observe other patients with multiple sclerosis, and do not know the contribution of her neurologic disease to this clinical appearance.

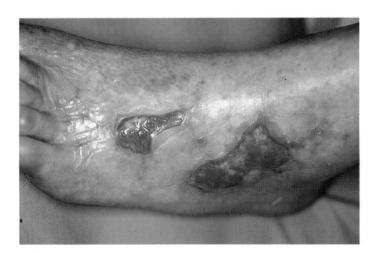

Figure 2.7
Fasciitis

This middle-aged man had eosinophilic fasciitis, which caused extensive fibrosis of his lower extremities. Distal pulses were barely detectable. We have been impressed by how difficult it is to detect arterial pulses in fibrotic extremities.

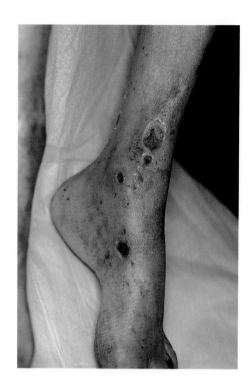

Figure 2.8a
Arterial ulcers

Note the normal contour of the leg and foot and the normal appearing epidermis in this female patient. The ulcers are punched out and necrotic. The patient was using potassium permanganate topically. We discourage the use of antiseptic solutions for the treatment of ulcers.

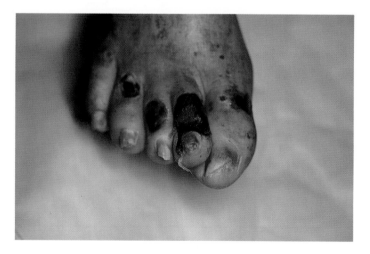

Figure 2.8b
Arterial ulcers/Close-up

Ulcers covered by eschars are also present on this patient's toes.

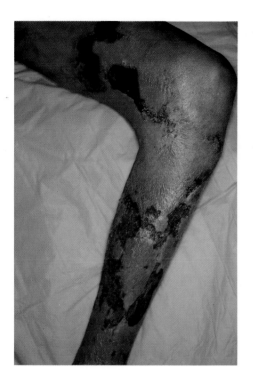

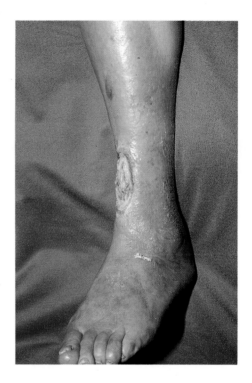

Figure 2.9
Atherosclerosis and ulceration

This clinical picture suggested a vasculitis or cholesterol embolization but biopsies failed to show evidence for these conditions. The patient died from other causes. An autopsy showed severe atherosclerosis. We have seen other cases in which large vessel atherosclerosis and ulcers such as these appear linked.

Figure 2.10
Arterial ulcer

The location and uniformly oval shape suggest the so-called "punched-out" arterial ulcer. The paradoxical erythema surrounding the ulcer probably results from endogenous vasodilatory substances, such as lactic acid, which are released in response to ischemia and hypoxia. Note also the often described absence of hair on this patient's leg and toes. As is typical, her pain was increased with leg elevation. Although she did not have a palpable pulse, it is not unknown for patients with severe reduction in arterial flow to have palpable pulses.

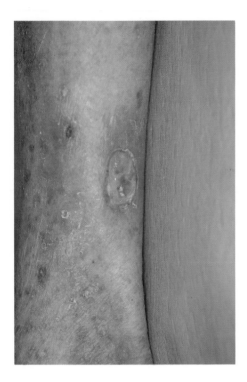

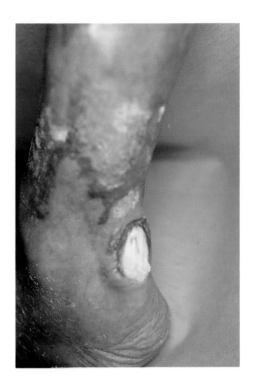

Figure 2.11
Arterial ulcer with a palpable pulse

This oval painful ulcer just superior to the Achilles tendon did not show evidence of cholesterol emboli histologically. The "reactive hyperemia" of arterial disease should not be misinterpreted either as cellulitis or as an indication of adequate blood flow. Angiograms showed definite obstruction even though her pulses were normal. Angioplasty was unsuccessful largely because her vessels could not be dilated and bled profusely. She died of a ruptured aortic thoracic aneurysm shortly after her unsuccessful surgery.

Figure 2.12
Cryofibrinogenemia

This woman with an ill-defined connective tissue disease has distal pulses that were quite feeble. This, and the presence of an exposed tendon, had suggested to her physicians that she might have arterial insufficiency. We were impressed by the purple and hemorrhagic lesions over the ankle. Both biopsies and plasma studies confirmed the diagnosis of cryofibrinogenemia.

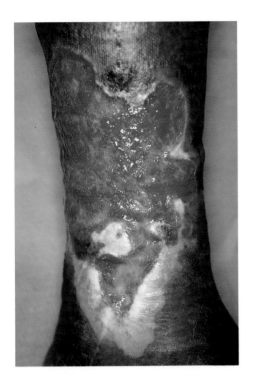

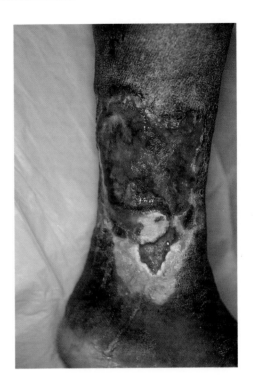

Figure 2.13a
Mixed arterial and venous ulcer in a patient with diabetes

This man's other leg had been amputated below the knee. This ulcer has not healed in spite of five years of therapy which included several grafting procedures. His arterial disease was inoperable. He walks with a prosthesis, crutches and this ulcerated limb. This patient's situation illustrates the complex nature of leg ulcers and leg ulcer therapy.

Figure 2.13b
Mixed arterial and venous ulcer in the same diabetic patient/Days later

The patient has had several such episodes where good granulation tissue, as seen in the previous illustration, is suddenly replaced by a necrotic and infected ulcer bed.

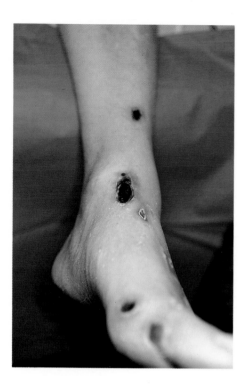

Figure 2.14
Arterial disease

A sudden onset of necrotic ulcers is not uncommon in patients with arterial disease. In this example there was no evidence histologically of vasculitis or cholesterol emboli. Arterial pulses were absent.

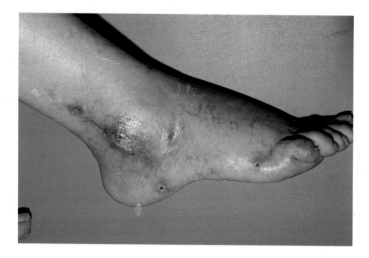

Figure 2.15
Antiphospholipid syndrome

Although the distal pulses were absent, vascular studies excluded the presence of arterial insufficiency. A biopsy from the ulcer edge showed intravascular thrombi in the dermis, and this female patient was found to have anticardiolipin antibodies. There was no evidence of systemic lupus erythematosus, which is often present in patients with this syndrome.

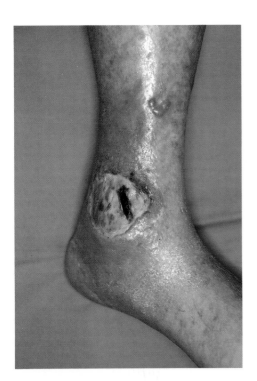

Figure 2.16a
Mixed venous and arterial ulcer

The necrotic tendon in the base of this ulcer strongly suggests that the ulcer is arterial. However, studies revealed that the extent of arterial insufficiency was limited. The man also had venous insufficiency, probably as a result of an injury and fracture of his ankle many years before.

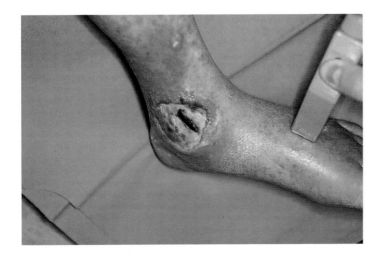

Figure 2.16b
Mixed venous and arterial ulcer/ Doppler sensor

Decreased blood flow was detected in this patient by Doppler examination. Normally, the ratio of systolic pressures in the foot to the arm is about 1.0. A ratio of 0.7 or less indicates arterial disease.

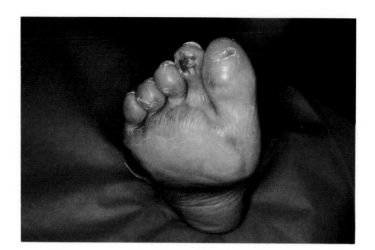

Figure 2.17
Cryofibrinogenemia

This 53-year-old man with leukemia was thought to have septic or cholesterol emboli. He had only slightly diminished pulses. The purpuric lesions and ulcers were finally found to be the result of cryofibrinogenemia.

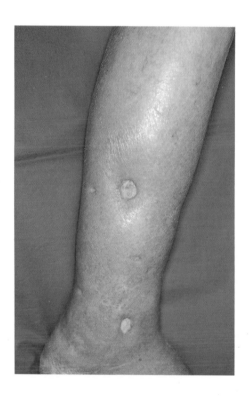

Figure 2.18
Candida infection

Because of the edema no leg pulses were detectable, even by Doppler, in this woman who was on systemic corticosteroid therapy for a connective tissue disease. Biopsy and culture of the ulcers showed infection with Candida. This situation illustrates the need for caution in deciding about the absence of pulses in swollen extremities.

3 Neuropathy

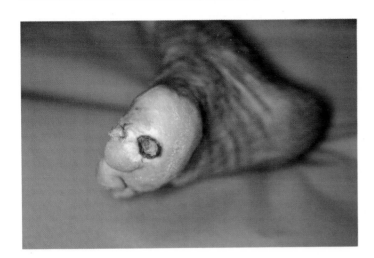

Figure 3.1a
Neuropathic ulcer in leprosy

This ulcer in this man with leprosy is at the junction of the great toe and plantar surface. The patient was applying gentian violet to the ulcer. This is a common location for ulcers in patients with an insensate foot.

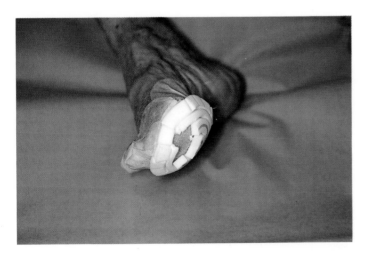

Figure 3.1b
Neuropathic ulcer in leprosy/ Treatment

Use of this modified pressure relieving dressing allowed the ulcer to heal.

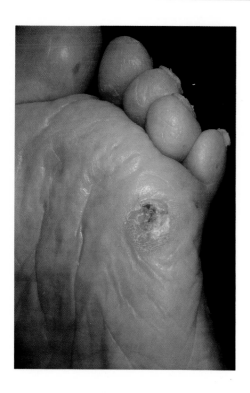

Figure 3.2
Foot of a diabetic

The callus over a metatarsal head is typical of diabetic pressure ulcers. This patient must stop bearing weight on this site.

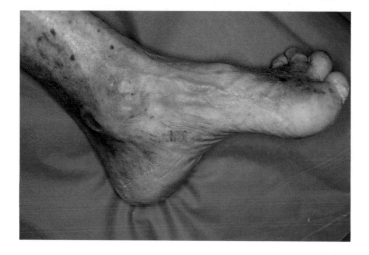

Figure 3.3
Venous ulcer in a male patient with leprosy

The deviated and distorted toes are part of the leprosy process. The ulcer's location forces one to consider venous ulceration. The patient had venous insufficiency demonstrated by photoplethysmography. A biopsy showed pericapillary fibrin and histologic changes of venous ulceration.

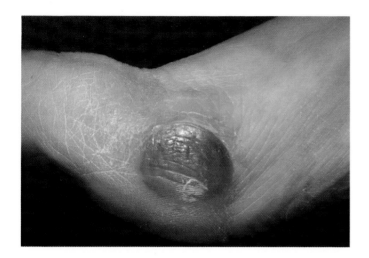

Figure 3.4a
Blistered foot of a diabetic

This blister is due to pressure on the metatarsal head. It could lead to ulceration.

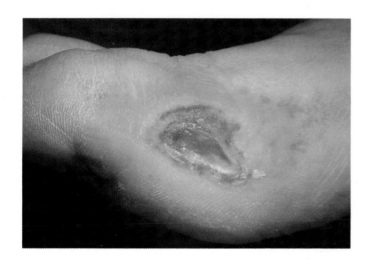

Figure 3.4b
Blistered foot of a diabetic/Follow up

This ulcer is healing rapidly. The patient is avoiding pressure and friction to the area.

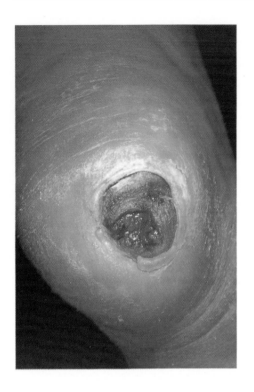

Figure 3.5
Diabetic ulcer of the heel

A large callus surrounds the ulcer of this male diabetic. The ulcer base is purple, suggesting imminent necrosis. As is often the case, he had osteomyelitis. The extent of tissue necrosis in pressure ulcers is usually much greater than what is suggested by the overlying epidermal defect.

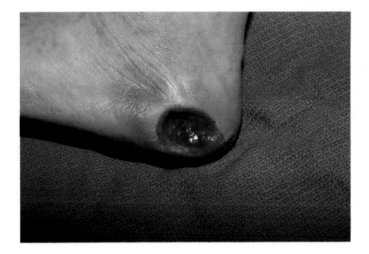

Figure 3.6
Diabetic heel ulcer after debridement

Diabetic pressure ulcers may have ample blood flow. The best results in such ulcers are obtained with vigorous surgical debridement and pressure avoidance.

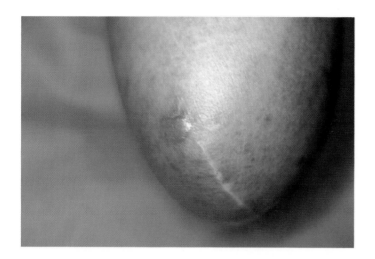

Figure 3.7
Blister on an amputation stump

This 63-year-old woman with diabetes and peripheral neuropathy had an amputation two years earlier. She periodically develops these blisters on the stump. The blisters are due to friction or pressure from the prosthesis and can lead to ulceration.

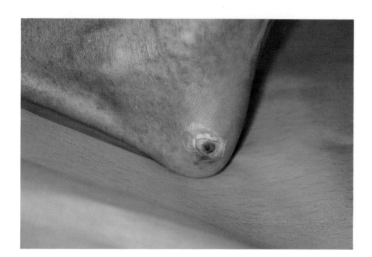

Figure 3.8
Pressure ulcer in diabetes

This is another example where it would be a mistake to judge the extent of necrosis from the size of the overlying skin defect. This female diabetic was found to have osteomyelitis.

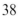

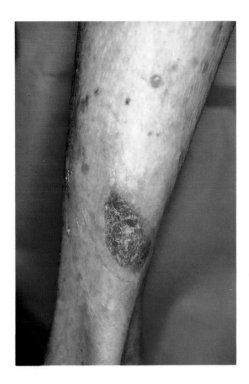

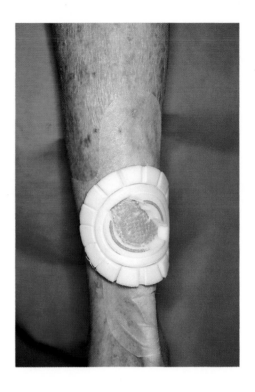

Figure 3.9a
Pressure ulcer in diabetes

This diabetic lady has a sensory neuropathy and is on hemodialysis. While undergoing dialysis she rests her legs on her recliner. Being insensate, she developed this ulcer at the site of sustained pressure.

Figure 3.9b
Pressure ulcer in diabetes/Treatment

Treatment with a composite pressure relieving occlusive dressing healed the ulcer.

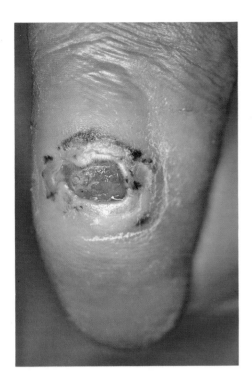

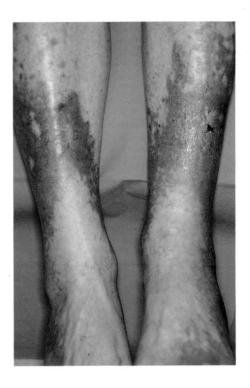

Figure 3.10
Neuropathic ulcer from leprosy/squamous cell carcinoma

This ulcer had been present for many years, but the bulging tumor-like process around the ulcer led us to do a biopsy which showed the presence of a squamous cell carcinoma.

Figure 3.11a
Neuropathy from frostbite

These pigment changes developed in this patient several months after a childhood bout of frostbite to both lower extremities. In the ensuing months he also developed hypesthesia and other evidence of neuropathy. All these cutaneous and neuropathic changes persisted in this 68-year-old man.

Continued

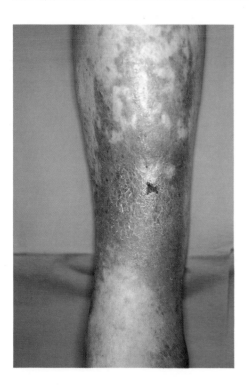

Figure 3.11b
Neuropathy from frostbite/Close-up

Note the hyperpigmentation over the shin.

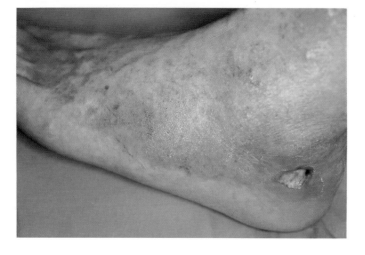

Figure 3.11c
Neuropathy from frostbite/ Ulceration

The patient has now developed an ulcer secondary to pressure near his heel.

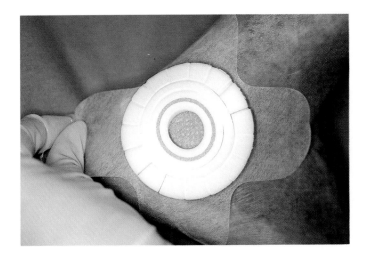

Figure 3.11d
Neuropathy from frostbite/Ulcer treatment

Use was made of a pressure relief dressing for the heel ulcer.

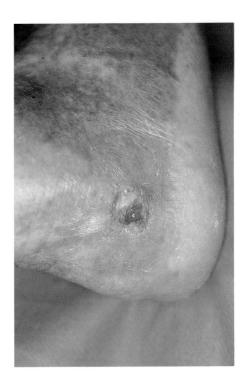

Figure 3.11e
Neuropathy from frostbite/Ulcer treatment

The patient responded well to pressure relief dressings.

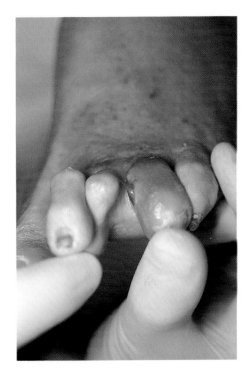

Figure 3.12a
Leprosy: ulcerated sausage-like toe

This pressure ulcer is due to excessive contact between these two toes.

Continued

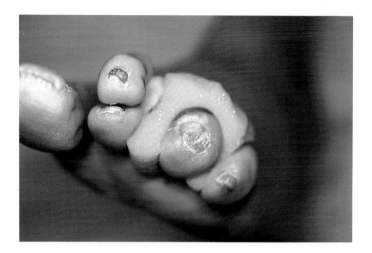

Figure 3.12b
Leprosy: ulcerated sausage-like toe/Ulcer treatment

The ulcer healed with relief of the pressure by a toe comb made of foam. The patient also used gentian violet. While topical antiseptics for ulcers are widely prescribed and may decrease the bacterial flora, their use may cause harm to the healing tissues. We discourage patients from using these agents.

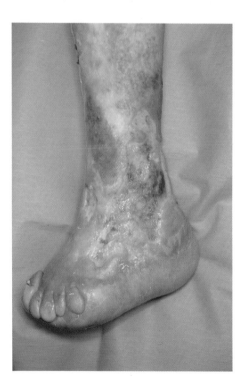

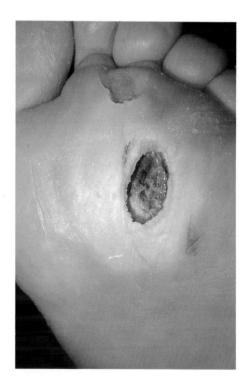

Figure 3.13
Leprosy

Resorption of the bones of the digits is more typical of leprosy than of diabetes. The cause of this woman's chronic ulcers is not clear although the tissues are free of mycobacteria.

Figure 3.14
Diabetic pressure ulcer

The extensive callus around this ulcer and undermined edges are characteristic of pressure ulcers. Experienced physicians trim away the callus and remove the underlying metatarsal head.

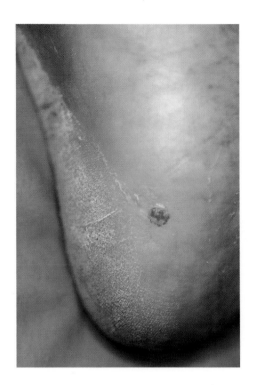

Figure 3.15
Sole ulcer

This tiny venous ulcer occurred as a satellite of a large venous ulcer on the leg (not seen in this photograph). Satellite venous ulcers are not uncommon but this location is extremely unusual. The patient had extensive vein stripping on that leg many years earlier. The satellite lesion was biopsied to rule out carcinoma. The patient did not have a neuropathy, and the ulceration is not surrounded by the callus typically seen in neuropathic ulcers.

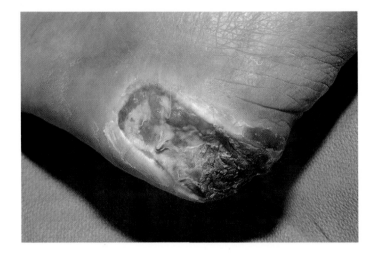

Figure 3.16
Osteomyelitis

It apparently took three or four weeks for this seriously infected ulcer to develop in this man with diabetes and foot neuropathy. Probing of the ulcer with a cotton applicator showed extremely friable tissues and easily exposed bones. He required amputation.

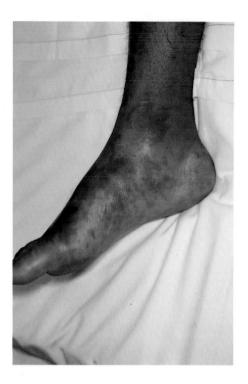

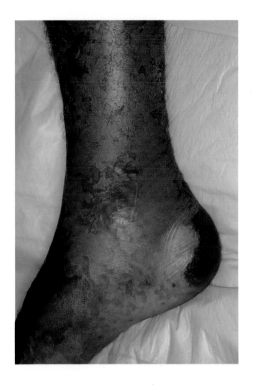

Figure 3.17a
Meningococcemia

Purpura of the lower extremities developed within hours in this 26-year-old man with meningococcemia. The purpuric lesions are irregular in shape, which suggests involvement of deep blood vessels.

Figure 3.17b
Meningococcemia/Pressure necrosis

Extensive necrosis of the heel developed within three days after hospitalization. This and similar cases have suggested to us that pressure necrosis may be more common in patients with vasculitis.

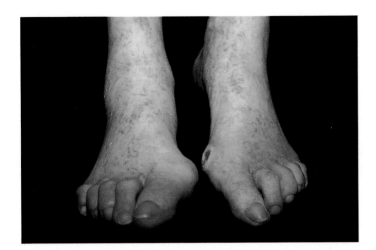

Figure 3.18
Diabetes and tight-fitting shoes

This is a clear example of how diabetic neuropathy combined with foot deformities and tight-fitting shoes can produce ulceration at pressure points. Patients with neuropathy and ulcers need periodic counseling and shoe adjustments to avoid pressure. It is important for patients to inspect their feet daily for signs of trauma.

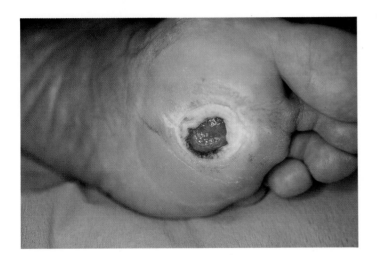

Figure 3.19
Diabetic metatarsal ulcer

The ulceration in this elderly man with diabetes and an insensate foot is a good example of callus formation at points of pressure. The deep and wide undermining is not apparent from the small epidermal ulcer surrounded by the callus. The ulcer should be probed and debrided. Extensive debridement is often needed.

Clinical points

- Ulcers are common in patients with rheumatoid arthritis and other connective tissue diseases

- Rheumatoid ulcerations have a "geographic" shape with smooth borders.

- Grafting of non-healing ulcers due to inflammatory conditions is often successful.

- Although biopsy of the ulcer bed and edge is helpful, especially in excluding other causes, pyoderma gangrenosum is generally diagnosed clinically.

- Pyoderma gangrenosum leads to considerable scarring upon healing.

- Pulse corticosteroid therapy is very effective in the treatment of pyoderma gangrenosum.

- Ulcers due to the antiphospholipid syndrome may heal with intralesional corticosteroid treatment.

- Stanozolol is a very effective treatment for ulcers due to cryofibrinogenemia.

- The application of retinoic acid to non-healing ulcers in immunocompromised patients promotes granulation tissue formation and healing.

- Atrophie blanche may be seen in many inflammatory and non-inflammatory conditions.

- Toe ulcers in patients with Raynaud's phenomenon and systemic sclerosis do not re-epithelialize readily but develop better granulation tissue with the use of occlusive dressings.

- Up to 20% of elderly patients with venous disease may have some degree of arterial insufficiency.

- Sudden widespread necrosis of the lower extremities may develop in patients with severe arterial insufficiency. The clinical picture may resemble periarteritis nodosa.

- Antiseptics should not be used in ulcers.

- Erythema surrounding arterial ulcers suggests reactive hyperemia.

- The sudden onset of livedo reticularis suggests cholesterol embolization.

- An ankle/arm systolic pressure ratio of 0.7 or less indicates arterial insufficiency.

- Ankle/arm systolic pressure ratios may give falsely normal readings in patients with diabetes mellitus and non-compressible arteries.

- Callus formation over a metatarsal head is typical of neuropathic pressure ulcers.

- Tissue necrosis in pressure ulcers is usually greater than suggested by the epidermal defect.

- Most diabetic ulcers are due to pressure. There is no evidence of "small vessel" obstructive lesions.

- Resorption of the bones of the digits is typical of leprosy.

- Patients with neuropathy and ulcers need periodic counseling and shoe adjustments to avoid pressure.

II SKIN AROUND THE ULCER

Introduction

In the preceding section, we stressed the need to "step back" and focus on the patient as a whole before making specific observations regarding the ulcer. This approach has made us aware of systemic problems that are intimately related to the ulceration or may even be its underlying cause. In this section we go to the next step, that is a careful observation of the tissue around the ulcer. We came to realize, as we gained more and more experience in diagnosing and treating leg ulcers, that we always (and almost subconsciously) looked for signs in the affected limb and around the border of the ulcer.

We have grouped the following subsections according to the following distinct clinical findings: atrophy, color and pattern changes, dermatitis, edema and induration. Each of these features tells a story and each becomes a guide to diagnosis, testing and treatment. Thus, a livedo-like pattern places the ulcer in the category of cholesterol embolization, cryofibrinogenemia, cryoglobulinemia, or antiphospholipid syndrome. Ulcers surrounded by indurated skin suggest the diagnosis of lipodermatosclerosis (as in venous ulceration), eosinophilic fasciitis and other dermal infiltrative processes. We learned to regard the diagnosis of venous ulceration with a high degree of suspicion when the ulcer did not have surrounding hyperpigmentation. Some features of the surrounding skin are almost diagnostic. The yellow atrophic skin of necrobiosis lipoidica diabeticorum is generally unmistakable. The hypertrophic overgrowth of lymphedema, the dermatitis of venous disease and the exquisite tenderness of cryofibrinogenemia are easily noted. We also found that certain clinical signs were not as helpful as had been generally stated. For example, we noticed that atrophie blanche, with its cold white atrophic lesions containing pinpoint red punctae, was rather non-specific and could be seen in a variety of inflammatory and non-inflammatory conditions.

Just as we cautioned the clinician not to miss the systemic problems in patients with leg ulcers, here we stress the need to pay close attention to what is around the ulcer. After a while, this approach becomes second nature.

4 Atrophy

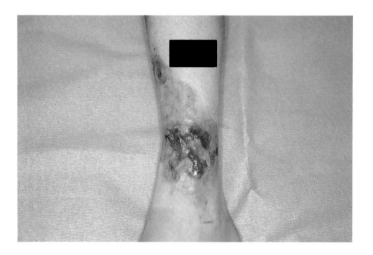

Figure 4.1
Necrobiosis lipoidica diabeticorum — ulcerated

The atrophy and yellow discoloration in combination with the ulceration in this location are all typical. Patients with necrobiosis lipoidica diabeticorum either have diabetes, will develop diabetes, or have a strong family history of diabetes.

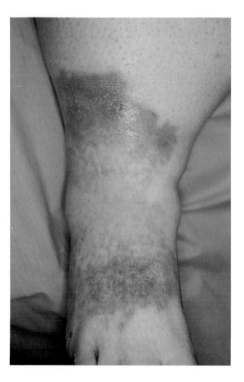

Figure 4.2
Necrobiosis lipoidica diabeticorum

The chronic use of topical corticosteroids to this lesion caused further atrophy and eventual ulceration.

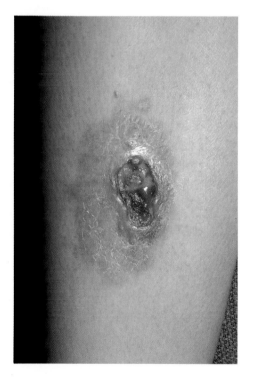

Figure 4.3
Ulcerated area of necrobiosis lipoidica diabeticorum

Once this teenage girl discontinued ice skating, her ulcerated shin lesion healed.

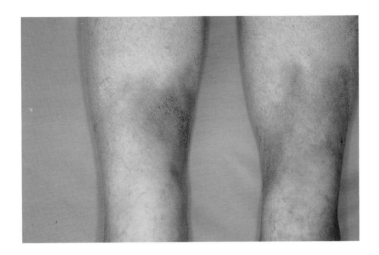

Figure 4.4
Acute and chronic lipodermatosclerosis

This photograph illustrates two different stages of lipodermato-sclerosis. The medial aspect of the right leg is intensely red; the skin is hard, may show a peau d'orange appearance, and the patient complaints of severe pain and tenderness. The left leg has already gone through this acute lipodermatosclerotic phase and has now entered the chronic phase of lipodermatosclerosis. The acute phase of lipodermatosclerosis responds dramatically to stanozolol treatment and to compression stockings.

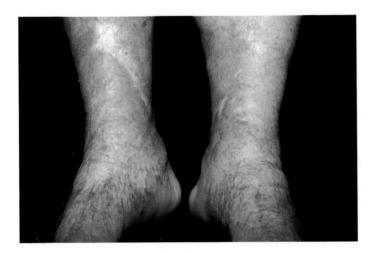

Figure 4.5
Lipodermatosclerosis and atrophie blanche

Areas of atrophie blanche and varicosities are particularly evident in this photograph. The skin is indurated. This combination of lipodermatosclerosis and atrophie blanche is not uncommon.

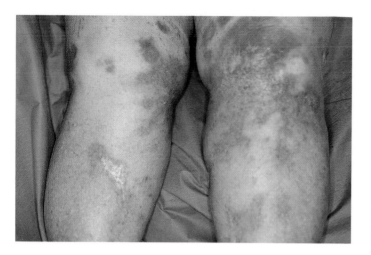

Figure 4.6
Atrophic changes in a diabetic

Occasional ulcerations complicated the course of this persistent eruption in a 63-year-old woman with diabetes. Histological features of necrobiosis lipoidica diabeticorum and granuloma annulare were present in different areas of this eruption. She had been treated with topical corticosteroids. As much as possible, we avoid topical corticosteroid treatment for lesions of lower extremities in diabetic patients. Such treatment can lead to skin atrophy and ulceration.

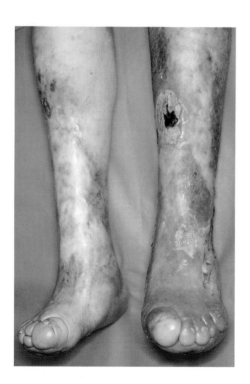

Figure 4.7
Leprosy

The resorption of the toes, as seen in this photograph, is accompanied by profound atrophy as well as fibrosis of the underlying tissues of the leg.

5 Color changes

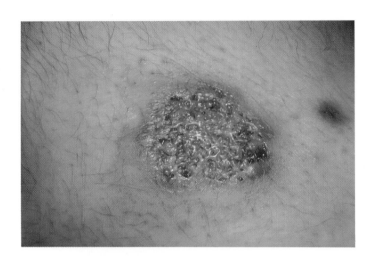

Figure 5.1
Pyoderma gangrenosum

The violaceous border as well as the cribriform surface are characteristic. The lesion in this female patient is healing following treatment with intravenous pulse corticosteroid therapy.

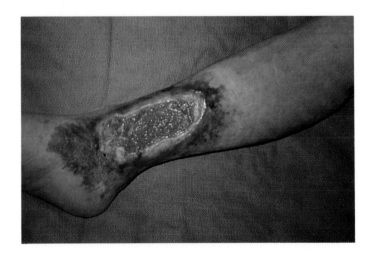

Figure 5.2
Exaggerated hyperpigmentation surrounding a venous ulcer

Biopsy showed hemosiderin deposition. There was no evidence of melanoma.

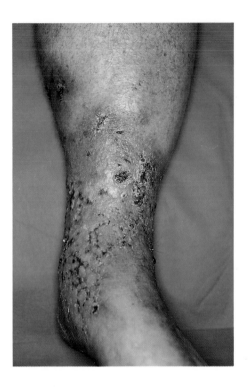

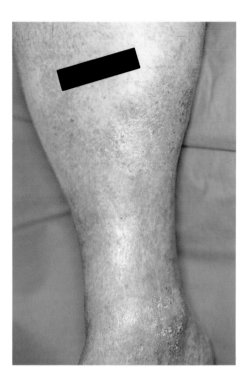

Figure 5.3a
Cryofibrinogenemia

This 69-year-old woman had a three-year
history of recurrent episodes of excruciatingly
painful lower extremity ulcerations. Other
physicians thought she had atrophie blanche or
vasculitis, and she had not responded to
pentoxifylline, aspirin, and dipyridamole (Per-
santine). She had partial responses to systemic
corticosteroids for short periods of time. The
significant features seen in this photograph are
the dusky, purple color of the lower leg with
erythema extending to the foot. There are many
areas of superficial skin necrosis of varying sizes.
The necrotic areas have a net-like appearance
on the medial aspect of her leg. The color of the
leg and the net-like configuration of the
ulcerations and necrosis are features strongly
suggestive of cryofibrinogenemia. In fact,
biopsies from these areas of ulceration failed to
reveal vasculitis but showed fibrin thrombi in
the dermis. She also had detectable levels of
plasma cryofibrinogen.

Figure 5.3b
Cryofibrinogenemia/Follow up

Two months of treatment with 6 mg/day of
stanozolol produced complete clearing of the
ulcerations seen in this photograph. The pain
was relieved after one to two weeks of
treatment. She did not have an underlying
systemic condition associated with cryofibrinogenemia.

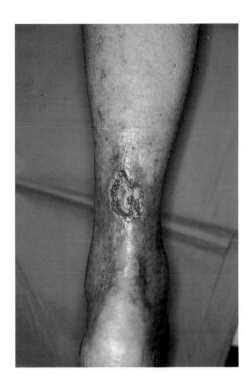

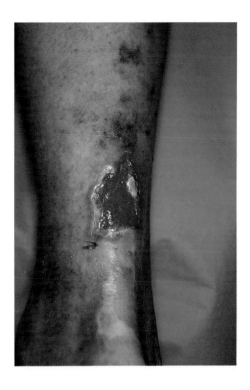

Figure 5.4a
Ulcer due to cryofibrinogenemia

This ulcer was present over the Achilles tendon
of this male patient. The exquisite pain, the
unusual location, the purple-red border, the
areas of necrosis and reticulate erythema with
pigmentation extending to the heel made us
consider the diagnosis of cryofibrinogenemia.
Biopsy showed fibrin thrombi and his plasma
was positive for cryofibrinogen. The cryofibrinogenemia was idiopathic.

Figure 5.4b
Ulcer due to cryofibrinogenemia/Treatment

After one month of stanozolol (6 mg/day) the
pain has disappeared. Healthy looking granulation tissue has developed within the ulcer, which
also shows evidence of reepithelialization.
However, new areas of necrotic skin are present
superior to the ulcer.

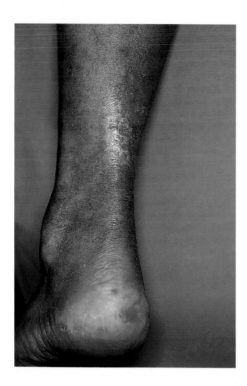

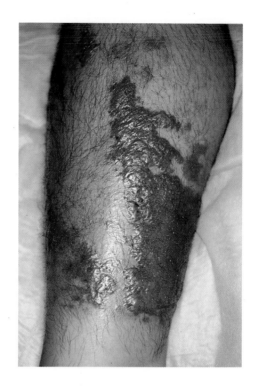

Figure 5.4c
Ulcer due to cryofibrinogenemia/Follow up

After three months of treatment with stanozolol the ulcer has completely healed and areas of necrosis are no longer present. However, the patient continues to have purple macules on the heel which have not ulcerated.

Figure 5.5
Unusual cellulitis

We have seen a number of patients with infection of the leg presenting as a vasculitis-like picture. We think that this is more a lymphangitis than a cellulitis. In this particular case characterized by high fever and constitutional symptoms, we were unable to determine the organism responsible for the infection. As in other similar cases, however, the patient required several weeks of systemic antibiotics to bring the infection under control.

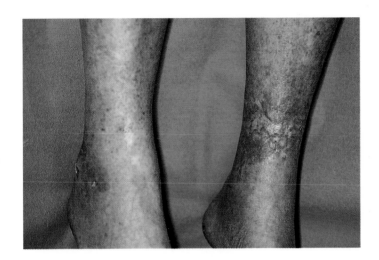

Figure 5.6a
Cryofibrinogenemia in a patient with leukemia

The lesions of atrophie blanche, the purple-red discoloration, and the punched-out and ragged edges all suggest the diagnosis in this man with chronic lymphocytic leukemia. There are ulcerations on both extremities.

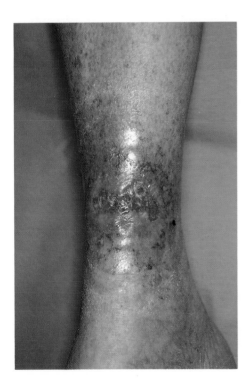

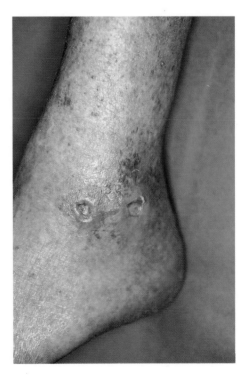

Figure 5.6b
Cryofibrinogenemia in a patient with leukemia/Follow up

The patient's pain was relieved and he ultimately healed with stanozolol treatment. Evidence of healing can be seen in this photograph.

Figure 5.6c
Cryofibrinogenemia in a patient with leukemia/Close-up

The white lesions of atrophie blanche, purpuric spots and violaceous erythema can all be appreciated in this photograph.

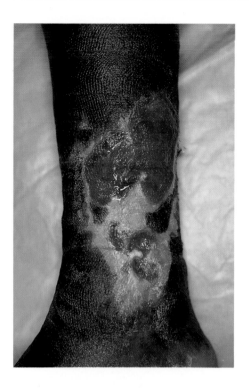

Figure 5.7
Mixed arterial and venous ulcer

The reepithelialized portions have not yet pigmented. Eventually pigmentation will occur.

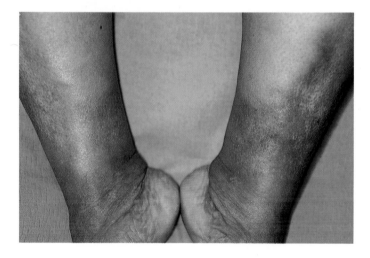

Figure 5.8
Chronic bilateral lipodermatosclerosis

The pigmentation and contour are characteristic.

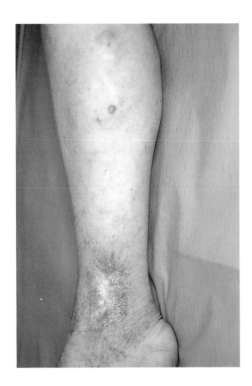

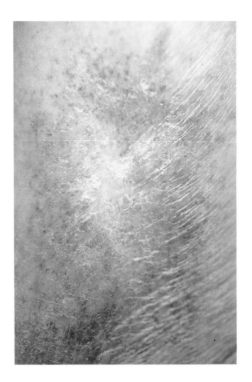

Figur 5.9a
Lipodermatosclerosis

This lady has discrete areas of lipodermatosclerosis. She also has obvious varicose veins.

Figure 5.9b
Lipodermatosclerosis/Close-up

The cold white lesions of atrophie blanche are
very common in venous disease.

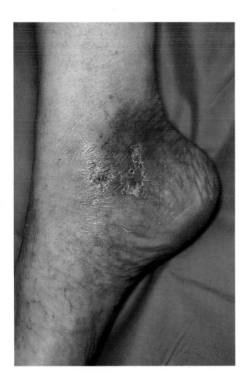

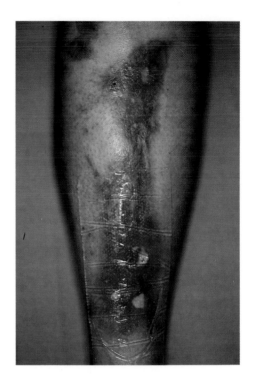

Figure 5.10
Painful malleolar ulcers

Although surrounded by hyperpigmented skin, this ulcer is not due to venous disease. The "angular" borders of this ulcer and the intractable pain suggested the diagnosis of ulceration due to intravascular fibrin thrombi. Some authors have labeled this entity livedoid vasculitis, although a vasculitis is not present. This female patient did not have cryoglobulinemia, cryofibrinogenemia, or the antiphospholipid syndrome. Malleolar ulcers from diverse etiologies tend to be disproportionately painful. Because these malleolar ulcers are so small the degree of pain the patients describe is hard to believe. This ulcer responded to stanozolol treatment.

Figure 5.11
Necrobiosis lipoidica diabeticorum

The yellow-red color of this condition is unmistakable. As in other similar cases we have observed, trauma seemed to be a precipitating event in the development of the ulcers. The gel dressing seen here was successful in relieving the pain.

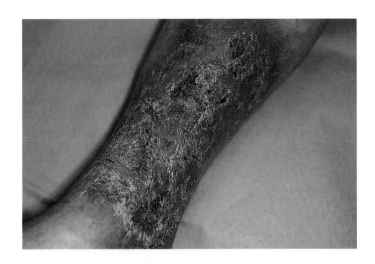

Figure 5.12a
Candida cellulitis

This acute episode of Candida cellulitis with erythema, pustules, scaling, and ulceration occurred in a female patient with chronic venous insufficiency and mottled pigmentation. KOH and culture were positive for Candida. The patient responded to treatment with oral ketoconazole.

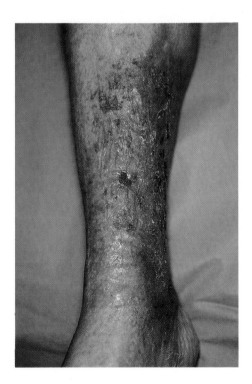

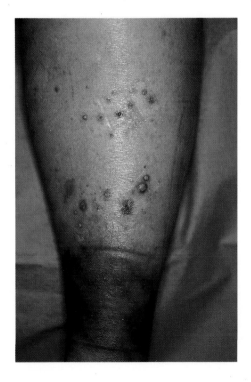

Figure 5.12b
Candida cellulitis/Follow up

Three weeks after ketoconazole treatment the ulcer healed.

Figure 5.13
Staphylococcal folliculitis

This infection developed beneath an Unna boot used to treat a venous ulcer in a patient with diabetes. Folliculitis and other infections beneath Unna boots are uncommon even in patients with diabetes.

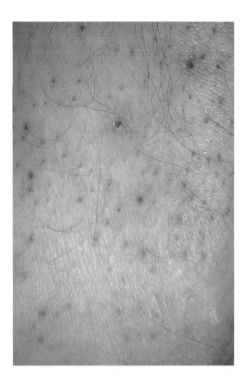

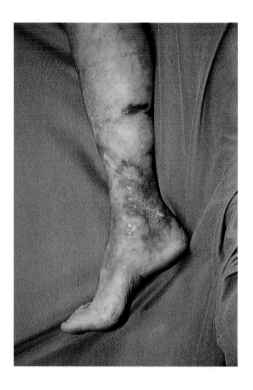

Figure 5.14
Scurvy

Follicular hemorrhage is seen in a patient with ascorbic acid deficiency and a non-healing venous ulcer. We also prescribe vitamin C in elderly patients with chronic ulcers.

Figure 5.15
Kaposi's sarcoma

This elderly man was thought to have "stasis" dermatitis. The linear growth on his calf is, however, very atypical for venous dermatitis. Biopsies confirmed our clinical suspicion of Kaposi's sarcoma.

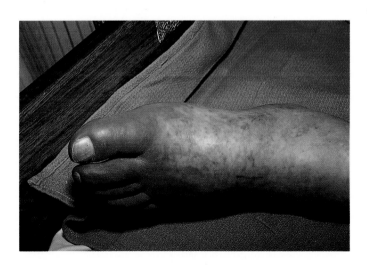

Figure 5.16
Disseminated intravascular coagulation (DIC)

The intensely purple toes of this man are cold and necrotic. A malignancy was the underlying cause of his DIC.

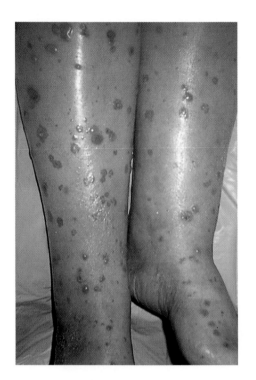

Figure 5.17a
Septic emboli

This woman with rheumatoid arthritis had a recent operation for total knee replacement and developed fever and these hemorrhagic blisters and pustules on her legs. Fluid from these vesicles grew *Staphylococcus aureus*, as did her blood cultures.

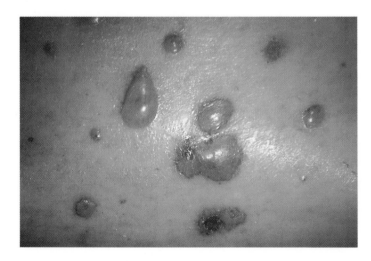

Figure 5.17b
Septic emboli/Close-up

Some of the lesions had ulcerated. This presentation of septic emboli is quite unusual.

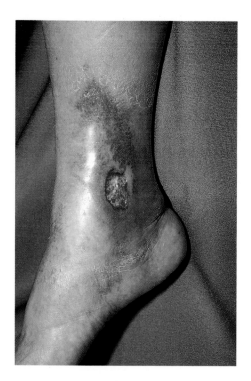

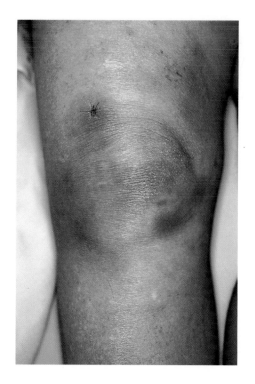

Figure 5.18
Ulcer within lipodermatosclerotic tissue

The color intensity of these brown and white indurated lesions is not common in lipodermatosclerosis. Ulcers tend to develop within this indurated skin.

Figure 5.19
Erythema nodosum

Painful red macules and plaques developed shortly after this woman received chemotherapy for a malignancy. The diagnosis of erythema nodosum was established by an excisional biopsy.

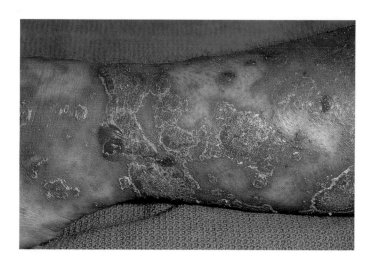

Figure 5.20
Lichen planus

This woman in her 50s developed lichen planus of the lower extremities after using thiazide diuretics. The purple-red color is characteristic of this condition, and the diagnosis was confirmed histologically. Erosions and ulcerations, as observed here, are uncommon in acute lichen planus.

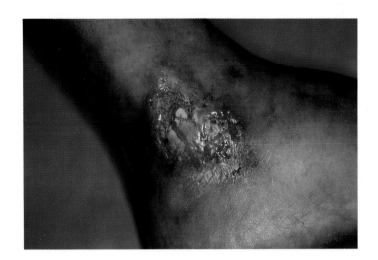

Figure 5.21
Ulcer associated with intravascular fibrin thrombi

The ankle ulcer in this 64-year-old man with severe diabetes and hypertension had not responded to topical therapy and occlusive dressings. The location argues against a neuropathic etiology and his pedal pulses were excellent. The necrotic wound bed, the purple edges, the livedo-like lesions on the leg suggest cryoglobulinemia, cryofibrinogenemia, cholesterol embolization, or the antiphospholipid syndrome. Blood tests for these diagnoses were negative but biopsy of the ulcer's edge showed intravascular fibrin deposition. Like other patients with this set of clinical and laboratory findings, he responded to stanozolol therapy.

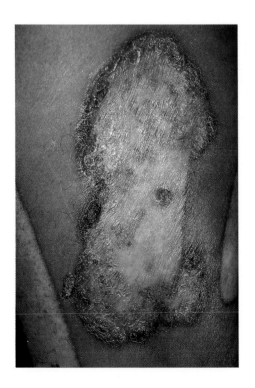

Figure 5.22
Pyoderma gangrenosum

The strikingly purple color of the jagged edges of the ulcer was the key to diagnosis in this man with diabetes. Although pyoderma gangrenosum is not generally associated with diabetes, we have seen a number of patients with this association. He responded to cyclosporin therapy.

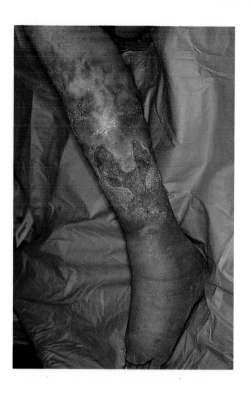

Figure 5.23a
Ulcers in a drug addict

This man in his 30s has a long history of intravenous drug addiction. He also injected drugs in the skin of his legs ("skin popping"). For the last two years he had lymphatic obstruction and venous disease with ulceration in his legs. The ulcer is highly exudative and is being treated with topical absorbing beads. Hyperpigmented "track marks" from his skin popping are seen in the upper part of this figure: they are quite typical.

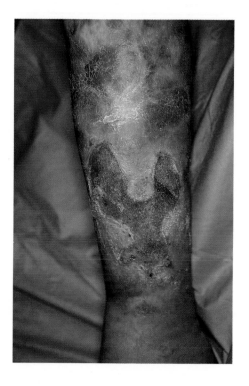

Figure 5.23b
Ulcers in a drug addict/Close-up

6 Dermatitis

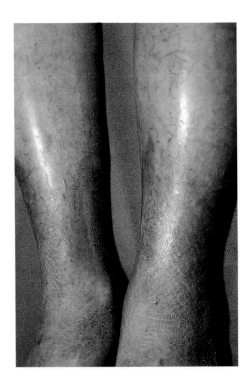

Figure 6.1
Severe xerosis

In people with venous, lymphatic, or arterial disease these fissures can lead to infection or ulceration.

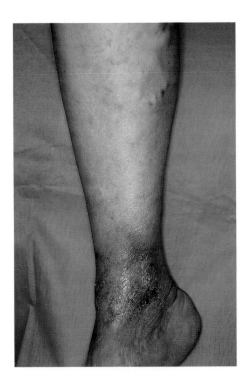

Figure 6.2
Venous disease

This photograph illustrates venous dermatitis around the gaiter area and large superficial veins in the calf.

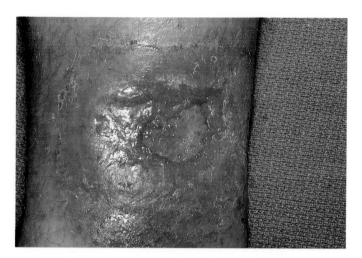

Figure 6.3
Venous ulcer and venous dermatitis

This dermatitis was restricted to the area beneath an occlusive dressing. This is uncommon; in fact, occlusive dressing therapy is often a useful treatment for venous dermatitis.

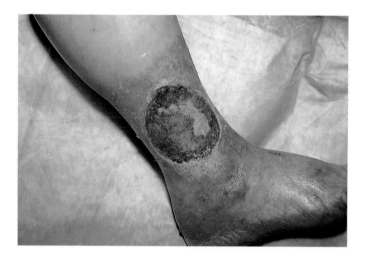

Figure 6.4
Venous ulcer and venous dermatitis

Acute dermatitis such as this has become rare in our leg ulcer population since we severely reduced our use of topical agents. Whenever possible, we choose systemic therapy over topical therapy for leg ulcers and the adjacent skin.

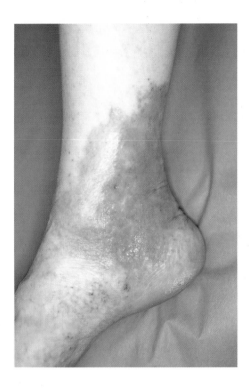

Figure 6.5
Contact dermatitis

This ulcer, which is almost healed, was being treated with neomycin topically.

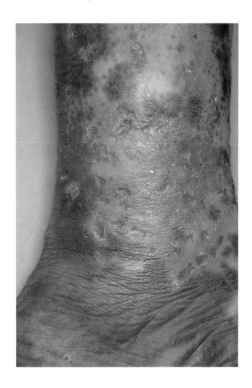

Figure 6.6
Healed excoriated ulcer

The healed ulcer of this man became pruritic. Unna boot treatment allowed these excoriations to heal. We often use the Unna boot to protect ulcers or dermatitis from exogenous agents.

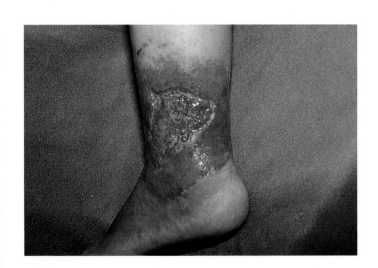

Figure 6.7
Venous ulcer with acute contact dermatitis

Patch testing documented several sensitivities in this woman. She became free of dermatitis by avoiding topical medications.

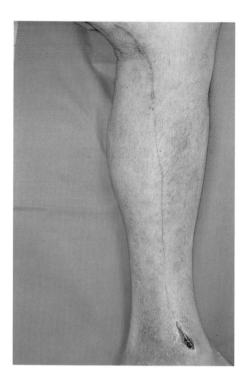

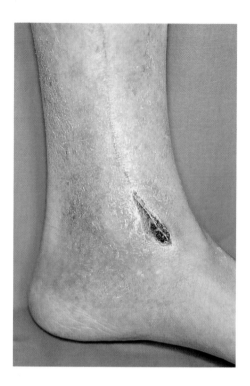

Figure 6.8a

Ulcer at the site of saphenous vein removal

Ulcers and dermatitis may develop within the surgical scar left by harvesting the saphenous vein. This is not uncommon.

Figure 6.8b

Ulcer at the site of saphenous vein removal/ Close-up

This ulcer healed after several weeks of compression therapy.

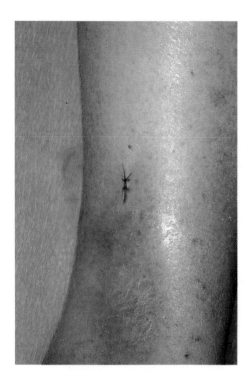

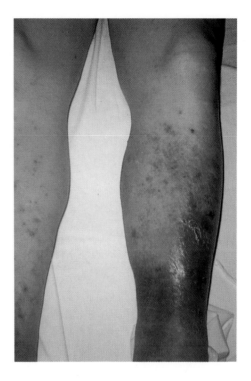

Figure 6.9
Lipodermatosclerosis/Signs of dermatitis

It is often not appreciated that the acute phase of lipodermatosclerosis is accompanied by substantial redness and scaling. These affected legs are also slightly edematous, which is probably responsible for the induration observed at this stage. Later on, in the chronic phase of lipodermatosclerosis, the induration is due to intense fibrosis and sclerosis of the underlying tissues. The photograph also illustrates the need for long and narrow excisional biopsies from the edge of the lesion when confirmation of the diagnosis is necessary. Punch biopsies in the center of this lipodermatosclerotic tissue could easily lead to a venous ulcer.

Figure 6.10
Contact dermatitis

A severe contact dermatitis was resolving from this lady's left leg, when red papules developed on her legs, palms and abdomen. Some have called this type of eruption "id reaction". The hyperpigmentation of her leg was due to longstanding venous disease.

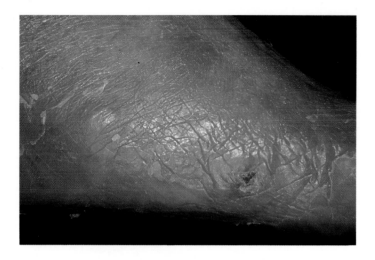

Figure 6.11
Scaling foot in an immunocompromised patient

For some time, this young man with a kidney transplant and taking cyclosporin A was thought to have a non-specific dermatitis of his foot. KOH and cultures showed a dermatophyte, which on biopsy of the tiny ulceration seen here was found to be invading the epidermis. His ulcer and dermatitis were cured with griseofulvin treatment.

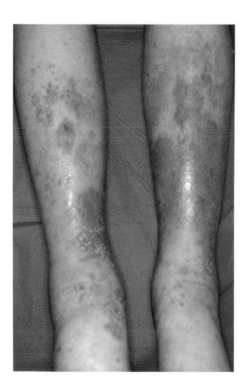

Figure 6.12
Psoriasis and venous disease

This woman with venous disease developed psoriasis in her 80s. The psoriatic plaques seemed to have a predilection for areas affected by venous disease.

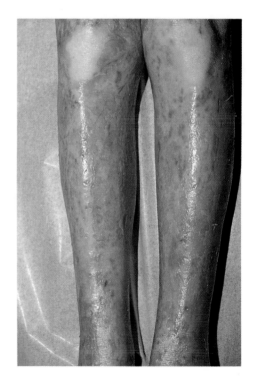

Figure 6.13
Pemphigus foliaceus

The erosions are the result of scratching and blistering from pemphigus. She responded very well to systemic corticosteroids.

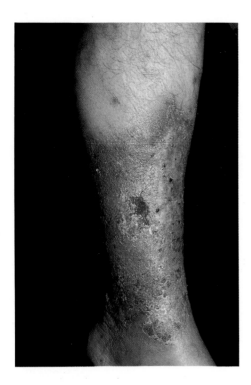

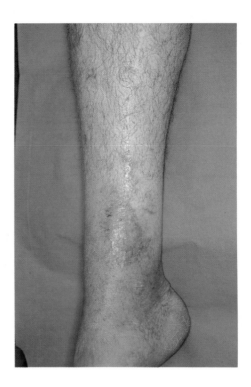

Figure 6.14
Ulcers and dermatitis

A chronic dermatitis was the major complica-
tion of venous disease in this elderly man. Ulcers
were frequently the result of scratching and
would heal easily with compression bandages.
The etiology of the dermatitis was not clear but
he reacted positively to several allergens. We
successfully treated him with 40 mg of oral
prednisone daily for three weeks, and this
therapy was tapered slowly over several weeks.
We prefer systemic to topical therapy in such
cases for fear of exacerbating the dermatitis with
topical medications.

Figure 6.15
"Saphenous" dermatitis

This man had his saphenous vein removed for
use in a coronary artery bypass procedure. He
developed this dermatitis along the course of the
donor site about a year later.

7 Edema

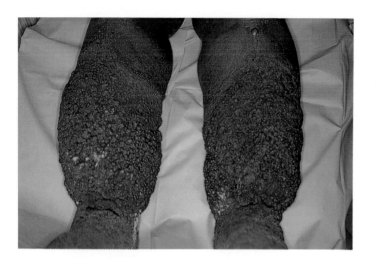

Figure 7.1a
Elephantiasis

This patient had normal looking legs a year earlier. We know that she developed an obstruction of the lymphatics due to enlarged lymph nodes in her abdomen. The etiology of her lymphadenopathy is unknown.

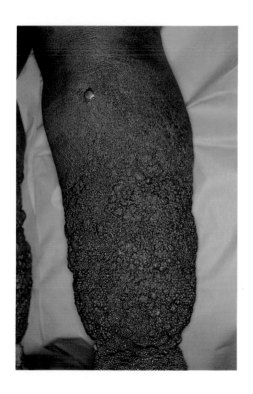

Figure 7.1b
Elephantiasis/Close-up

Biopsy of these lesions showed epithelial hyperplasia and fibrosis. Polymerase chain reaction for several papilloma viruses was negative.

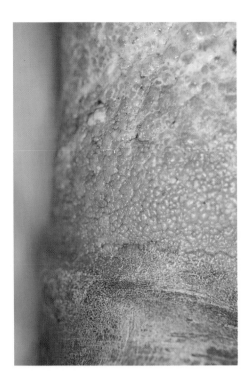

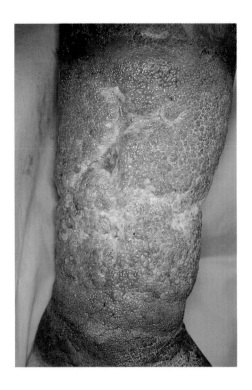

Figure 7.2a
Lymphedema

This is an excellent example of the pebbly appearance of lymphedematous skin, which shows epithelial hyperplasia histologically.

Figure 7.2b
Lymphedema/Ulcer

These limbs are most often foul smelling. Ulceration is not uncommon with lymphedema. Compression is an important component of treatment.

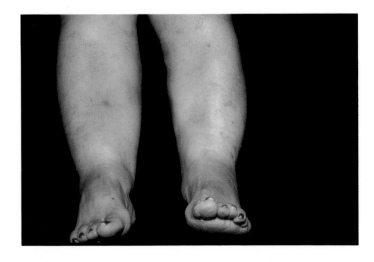

Figure 7.3
Bilateral lymphedema

The tubular configuration of these legs is distinct.

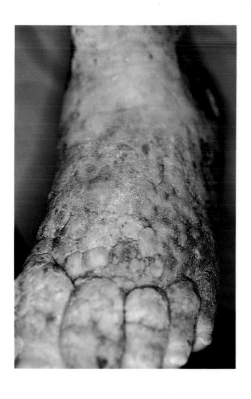

Figure 7.4
Lymphedematous foot

Patients with this condition may also suffer from recurrent leg cellulitis. Often treatment with systemic or topical antifungal agents is necessary to prevent toe web fissures which are presumed to be portals of entry for the bacteria that cause the cellulitis. In some cases prophylactic treatment with antistaphylococcal agents is necessary.

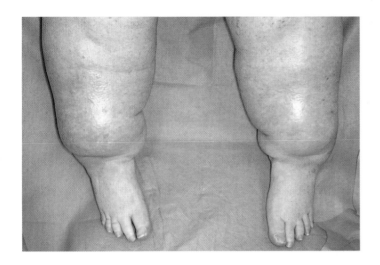

Figure 7.5a
Congenital lymphedema—Milroy's disease

This female patient has had this condition for over 40 years, as has her sister. There is no swelling of her feet.

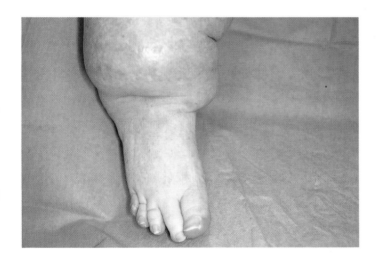

Figure 7.5b
Congenital lymphedema—Milroy's disease/Close-up

Obesity has been reported as a cause of similar appearing enlarged lower extremities sparing the feet.

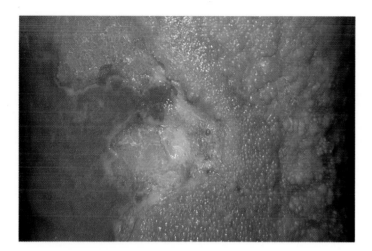

Figure 7.6
Verrucous hyperplasia at the edge of a venous ulcer

This change indicates lymphatic obstruction.

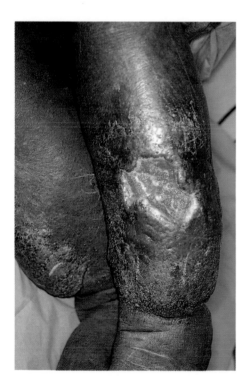

Figure 7.7
Ulcer due to lymphedema

Another example of massive longstanding lymphatic obstruction with ulceration. The cause of the lymphedema is unknown.

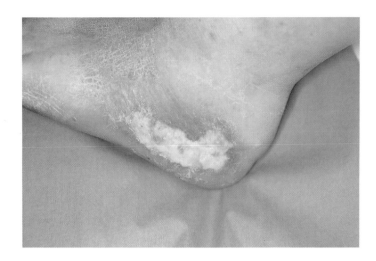

Figure 7.8
Squamous cell carcinoma and lymphedema

This nurse developed fibrosis and lymphedema of the entire limb after self injection of Talwin into the thigh and lower extremity. The lateral sole area ulcerated repeatedly. The extent of thickened stratum corneum seen here as white hydrated material is unusual. Carcinoma was finally diagnosed from a large biopsy at the ulcer's edge near the heel.

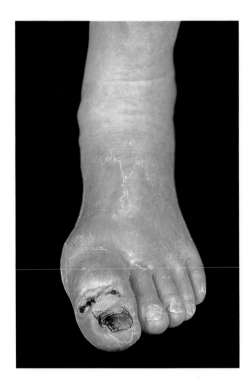

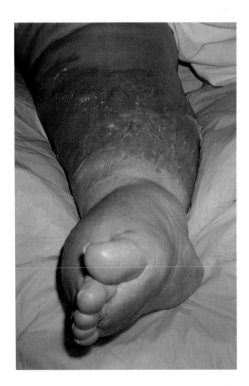

Figure 7.9
Cellulitis

This edematous foot and cellulitis developed after a chemical burn.

Figure 7.10a
Erysipelas

The red vesicular process skips the foot and starts at the ankle. This is not uncommon with erysipelas, a lymphangitis. In cellulitis, an infection of the subcutaneous tissues, the involvement is more diffuse and less well demarcated.

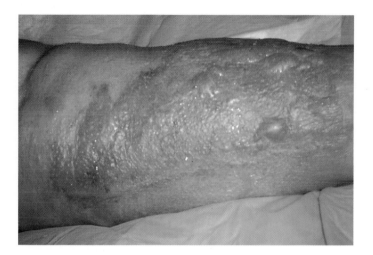

Figure 7.10b
Erysipelas/Dermatitis-like process

Note the vesicular and hemorrhagic involvement of the anterior portion of the leg. Due to invasion of lymphatics, the skin involvement is extremely well demarcated. Because of this dramatic feature, the physician who first evaluated this patient misdiagnosed the condition as contact dermatitis. She eventually responded completely to intravenous antibiotics.

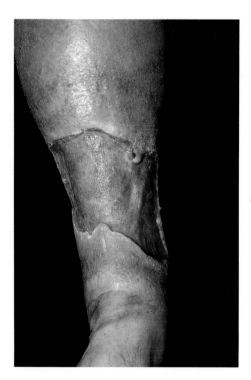

Figure 7.11
Large ulcer

This woman had evidence of both venous (by photoplethysmography) and lymphatic disease (by lymphangiography), a not uncommon combination.

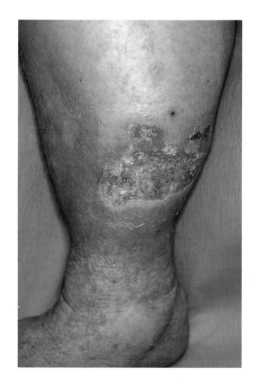

Figure 7.12
Lymphedema and venous disease

Massively enlarged legs often develop in patients with venous disease complicated by lymphatic damage. The ulcer is longstanding, but biopsies have not shown evidence of cancer.

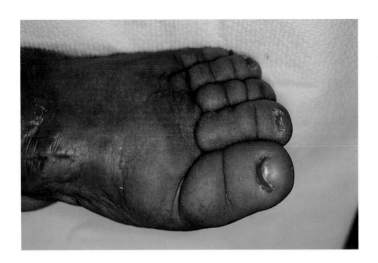

Figure 7.13
Cellulitis

This lady was being treated for a venous ulcer when her toes became swollen and warm. She responded to intravenous antibiotics. This degree of toe swelling is distinctly unusual in patients with uncomplicated venous ulcers.

8 Induration

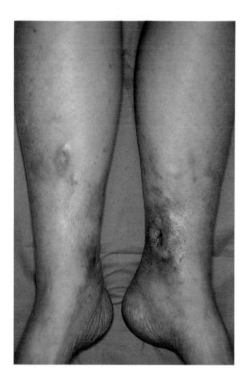

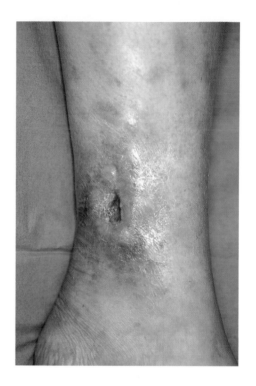

Figure 8.1a
Ulceration within areas of nodular amyloidosis

A biopsy of the edge of this ulcer showed amyloid deposits. The raised lesions suggest a dermal process. This patient illustrates the value of biopsying ulcerations. Initially, the location and clinical features of the ulcer strongly suggested venous disease but the patient did not improve with leg compression therapy.

Figure 8.1b
Ulceration within areas of nodular amyloidosis/Close-up

The hyperpigmentation is similar to that observed in venous disease, and the area also displayed the same type of induration observed in lipodermatosclerosis.

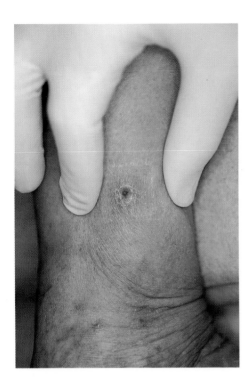

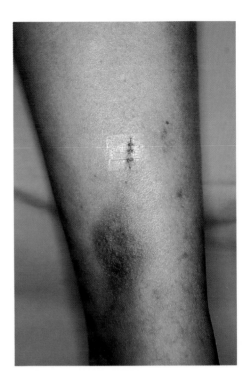

Figure 8.2
Slow healing punch biopsy in the center of an area of lipodermatosclerosis

Lipodermatosclerotic skin is indicated here by the inability of the physician to compress the tissues. Biopsies of lipodermatosclerosis are often difficult to heal and about half of the time become ulcers. When a biopsy is necessary, we biopsy lipodermatosclerosis near the edge of the indurated area rather than in the center, since biopsies of the edges of venous ulcers surrounded by lipodermatosclerosis seem generally to heal without difficulty.

Figure 8.3
Biopsy of lipodermatosclerosis

We show this as another example of the type of biopsy we prefer to perform in such patients to prevent wound dehiscence and the development of an ulcer at the biopsy site. The long and narrow incision is made at the margin of indurated tissue, which is ascertained by careful palpation.

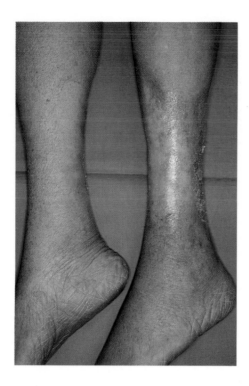

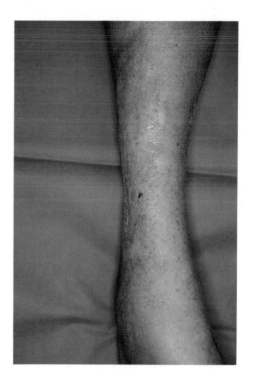

Figure 8.4a
Lateral lipodermatosclerosis

The inverted "bowling pin" shape of both legs is seen clearly. The shiny, fibrotic and bound-down appearing skin on the lateral side of both legs is in sharp distinction to the medial skin on both legs which is not atrophic, not bound-down and not hard and shiny.

Figure 8.4b
Lateral lipodermatosclerosis

The lateral side has epidermal atrophy (a shiny surface), some ill defined erythema, and a small crusted erosion. The medial side appears normal. This presentation of lateral lipodermatosclerosis must be exceedingly rare.

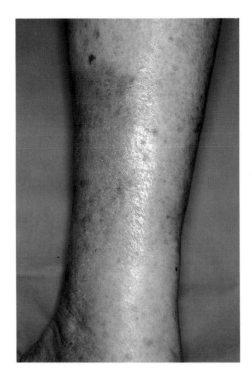

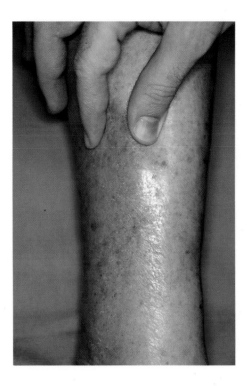

Figure 8.5a
Acute phase of lipodermatosclerosis

This mildly red lesion is quite painful and tender. It is often not recognized or is misdiagnosed as a cellulitis.

Figure 8.5b
Acute phase of lipodermatosclerosis/Close-up

Although not appreciated photographically, the area is indurated and bound-down. The attempts to pinch the tissue between the thumb and forefinger illustrate the thickened nature of this skin. The acute phase of lipodermato-sclerosis may last weeks or months. It can be improved dramatically with compression ther-apy, stanozolol treatment (4–6 mg/day), or both. The acute phase is often followed by a chronic phase characterized by lack of pain and severely bound-down skin. Ulcers frequently develop within the lipodermatosclerotic skin.

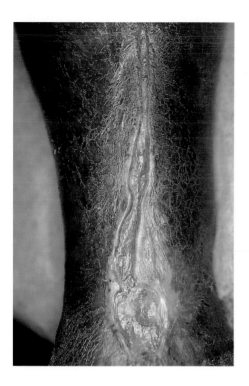

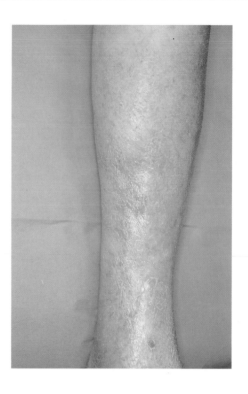

Figure 8.6
Venous disease

This patient has a typical venous ulcer near the
ankle. The lipodermatosclerosis extends to the
top of the photograph. The linear extension of
the ulcer appears almost as though an area of
intense lipodermatosclerosis had lost its tensile
strength.

Figure 8.7
Lipodermatosclerosis

The redness of the acute phase has almost
disappeared, as has the pain. The lesion is on its
way to becoming chronic lipodermatosclerosis.

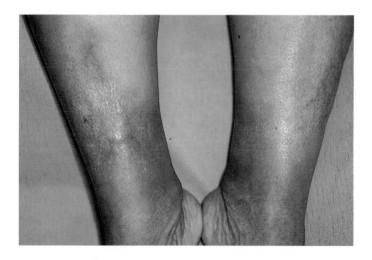

Figure 8.8
Bilateral lipodermatosclerosis

These hyperpigmented areas are
hard and non-tender. Ulcers may
develop within these lesions upon
even minor trauma.

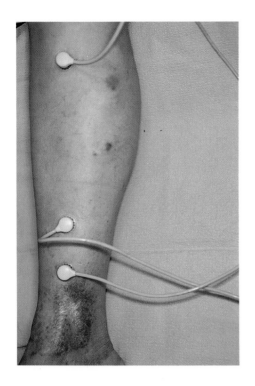

Figure 8.9
Healed venous ulcer in an area of lipodermatosclerosis

In this healed venous ulcer the area of atrophie blanche is especially large, covering most of the central portion of the healed ulcer, which is intensely lipodermatosclerotic. Sensors for transcutaneous oxygen measurements placed at decreasing distances from the healed ulcer detect progressively reduced levels of oxygen tension.

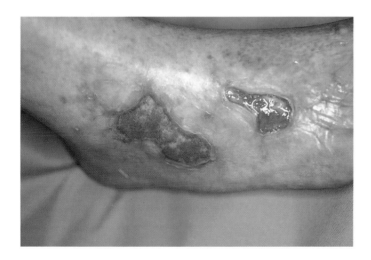

Figure 8.10a
Eosinophilic fasciitis

These foot ulcers in this man with eosinophilic fasciitis have proved very difficult to heal. This is often the case with ulcers in fibrotic skin.

Continued

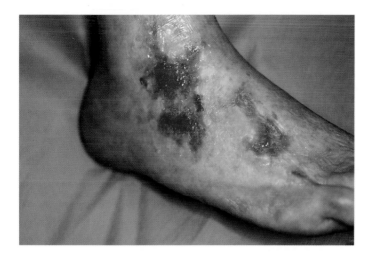

Figure 8.10b
Eosinophilic fasciitis/Follow up

Some reepithelialization was obtained with the use of foam dressings. These synthetic dressings provide a moist environment but do not adhere to the healing skin.

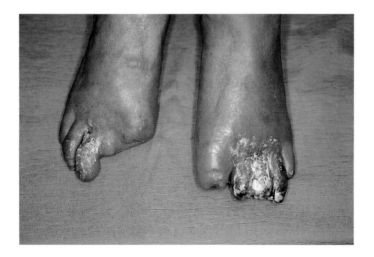

Figure 8.11
Autoamputation/systemic sclerosis

One by one these digits have become gangrenous and autoamputated. This female patient is being treated with topically applied silver sulfadiazine cream. Whenever gangrene occurs in patients with systemic sclerosis, the possibility of an upstream thrombus must be excluded.

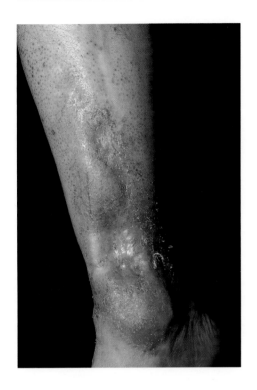

Figure 8.12a
Chronic osteomyelitis

This 60-year-old man had a bullet injury to his leg 20 years ago, followed by a chronic ulceration and osteomyelitis at the site. Despite many intensive courses of antibiotic treatment and surgeries, the osteomyelitis persisted. The long and protracted course has produced fibrosis and scarring. Some areas around the ulceration appear atrophic and others are hypertrophic.

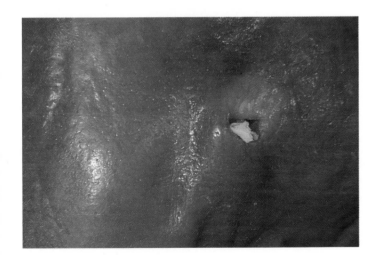

Figure 8.12b
Chronic osteomyelitis/Close-up

Just above the medial malleolus, a small ulceration is still present which is seen packed with gauze. This is an example of the fact that osteomyelitis can be present many years after the initial injury.

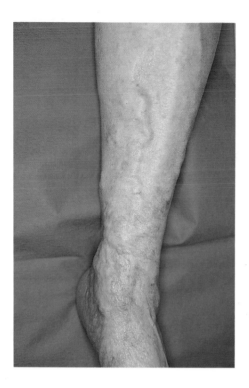

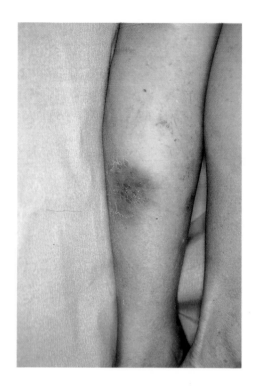

Figure 8.13
Varicose veins

By themselves varicose veins do not predict the development of venous ulcers. This female patient has had these varicose veins for many years. The absence of skin induration, which is a hallmark of lipodermatosclerosis, portends a good prognosis in terms of ulcer development. It is a minority of patients who develop venous ulcers without first going through a lipodermatosclerotic stage.

Figure 8.14
Suppurative panniculitis

This painful lesion developed suddenly in this 43-year-old woman with ulcerative colitis. It is red, scaling, and indurated. The location argues strongly against the diagnosis of lipodermatosclerosis. A full-thickness biopsy showed a suppurative panniculitis.

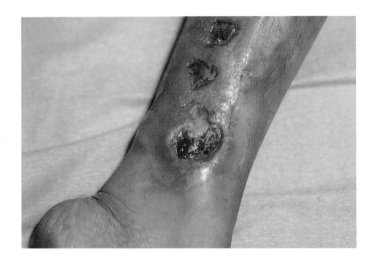

Figure 8.15a
Silicone injections

More than 20 years after having her legs injected with a silicone containing preparation for cosmetic reasons, this 42-year-old woman developed ulcers within the injected areas. The skin was hard and tender. Histologically, an intense inflammatory infiltrate and numerous clear vacuoles were present in the dermis and subcutaneous tissue. We have seen patients with complications ranging from minor discomfort to fasciitis and ulceration.

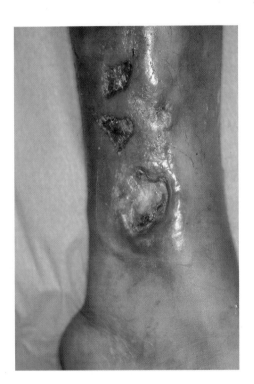

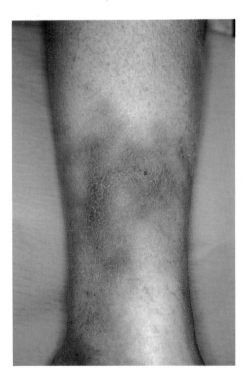

Figure 8.15b
Silicone injections/Follow up

The patient healed with a combination of occlusive dressings and oral antiinflammatory agents, including antimalarials and corticosteroids.

Figure 8.16
Acute lipodermatosclerosis

This is a very painful condition. The patient was misdiagnosed as having morphea and cellulitis by other physicians. The pain was largely gone after two weeks of stanozolol treatment.

Clinical points

- The chronic use of topical corticosteroids on the lesions of necrobiosis lipoidica diabeticorum may cause further atrophy and eventual ulceration.

- A necrotic ulcer bed with a surrounding livedo pattern suggests that the ulcer may be due to occlusion of small blood vessels by cryoproteins or thrombi.

- Patients with ulcers due to cryofibrinogenemia do not generally worsen with cold exposure.

- Cryoglobulins are measured in serum, whereas cryofibrinogen is measured in plasma.

- Newly re-epithelialized skin is hypopigmented. It takes several months for pigment to develop.

- The cold white lesions of atrophie blanche are very common in venous disease.

- Folliculitis and other infections are unusual beneath Unna boots and other compression bandages.

- Many older people have low vitamin C levels. Give vitamin C to elderly patients with non-healing ulcers.

- Venous dermatitis is exceedingly rare in patients who avoid topical preparations. Whenever possible we choose systemic therapy rather than topical therapy for leg ulcers and the adjacent skin.

- Venous ulcers frequently develop or recur within lesions of lipodermatosclerosis.

- Ulcers and dermatitis may develop within the surgical scar left by harvesting the saphenous vein.

- The acute phase of lipodermatosclerosis, also known as hypodermitis sclerodermiformis or sclerosing panniculitis, is accompanied by intense pain, erythema and scaling. It responds dramatically to stanozolol.

- Legs affected by primary lymphedema are swollen and have a tubular configuration. Typically, the feet are spared.

- Reduced lymphatic drainage is common in venous disease. Verrucous hyperplasia at the edge of venous ulcers may indicate a component of lymphatic obstruction.

- Squamous cell carcinoma may develop within long-standing ulcers.

- Biopsies of lipodermatosclerosis should be done by thin excision (closed primarily) at the edge of the lesions. Punch biopsies from the center of lipodermatosclerosis may not heal.

- Lipodermatosclerosis is almost always more pronounced on the medial aspect of the leg.

- Whenever toe gangrene occurs in patients with systemic sclerosis, the possibility of an upstream thrombus must be excluded.

III ULCER BED

Introduction

In the previous two sections we have shown several examples of how much information about the ulcer is gained by paying attention to systemic features and the condition of the skin surrounding the ulceration. Indeed, by the time the ulcer bed becomes the intellectual focus of our exam, we should have a fairly reasonable idea of the ulcer etiology. For example, we may know by now that the patient has lipodermatosclerosis and is thus likely to suffer from a venous ulcer. By this time we should definitely know whether the ulcer is secondary to necrobiosis lipoidica diabeticorum. The absence of arterial pulses, the presence of a neuropathy, evidence of lymphatic obstruction are already known by now.

Indeed, with a few exceptions, the information gained from examining the ulcer bed is generally less specific than that obtained thus far. Those exceptions, however, are notable. For example, the presence of an eschar and dark necrotic tissue implies arterial occlusion, either from atherosclerosis or from vasculitis or cryoproteins. Venous ulcers neither have this type of necrotic ulcer bed nor do they show necrotic tendons. However, a superficial fibrinous or "gelatinous" necrosis may occur suddenly in venous ulcers. Another example of the usefulness of closely examining the ulcer bed is the clinical recognition of basal cell carcinoma in an ulcer. These tumors often look like exuberant granulation tissue growths within the ulcer bed. We will discuss how the glistening nature of these tumors and other features of the ulceration will point to the right diagnosis.

Another clue offered by a thorough exam of the ulcer itself is undermining of the edges and the fenestrated pattern of ulceration which is often seen in pyoderma gangrenosum. The shape of the ulcer, too, will be helpful in diagnosis. Punched out ulcers are more typical of arterial occlusion, pressure or primary infectious processes. Venous ulcers and pyoderma gangrenosum tend to have an irregular shape. In general, however, many other features of the ulcer bed are less specific. Malodor, exudation, poor granulation tissue and minimal dermal necrosis are all seen in most types of ulcers.

Debridement is important in ulcer management. In addition to using occlusive dressings to obtain a painless autolytic debridement, surgical, enzymatic and fixative methods may be used. Exudation is often induced by occlusive dressing therapy, especially in the early stages of treatment. Although the exudate under occlusive dressings is often malodorous and yellow/brown, it does not indicate infection. Hypertrophic granulation tissue may be secondary to occlusive dressing therapy. Contrary to what is generally thought, good granulation tissue does not always result in epithelialization. This is especially the case with venous ulcers.

9 Calcifications

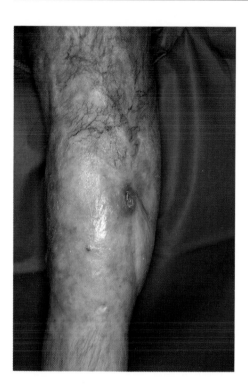

Figure 9.1a
Ulceration secondary to dystrophic calcification

This man burned his leg many years ago. The ulcer contains chunks of calcified tissue. Conservative therapy with occlusive dressings and topical agents failed. The ulcer healed completely after wide surgical debridement.

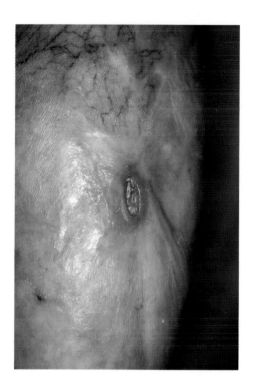

Figure 9.1b
Ulceration secondary to dystrophic calcification/Close-up

The ulcer base is made of calcified material.

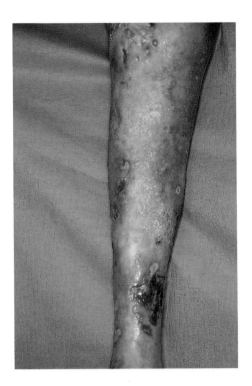

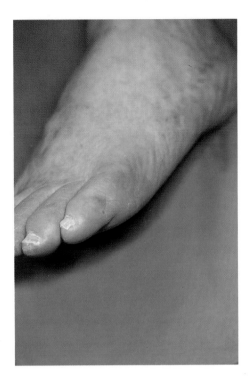

Figure 9.2
CREST syndrome

This female patient has extensive leg fibrosis and calcinosis with multiple ulcerations. The ulcer bases are formed of calcified tissue.

Figure 9.3
Calcinosis responding to warfarin

This woman with systemic sclerosis was suffering from an intensely painful area of calcinosis on the lateral aspect of the fifth metatarsal. This red area was extremely tender to the touch, and she was incapacitated to the point that she could hardly walk. Low doses of warfarin have been used successfully for this otherwise recalcitrant condition. Within a month of starting therapy with 2.5 mg/day of warfarin, the redness subsided and she was able to walk with much less pain.

10 Debridement

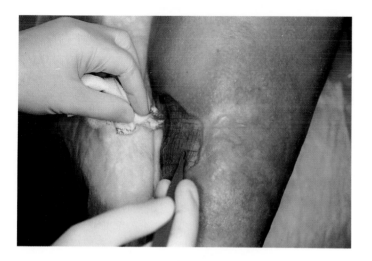

Figure 10.1a
Arterial ulcer — method of debridement

This arterial ulcer was covered by firm necrotic material. The ulcer base has been repeatedly incised with a scalpel in a checkerboard fashion. This is a painless procedure because the wound bed is necrotic.

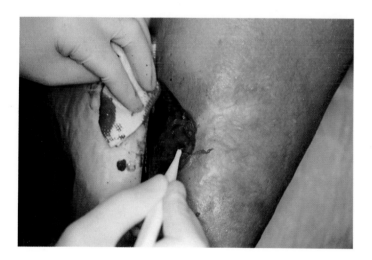

Figure 10.1b
Arterial ulcer — method of debridement/Continued

Incision in this checkerboard fashion facilitates curettage because it frees each square from the surrounding tissue. The squares are easily curetted from their connection at the base. This method avoids pulling on the surrounding tissues, which would have been painful.

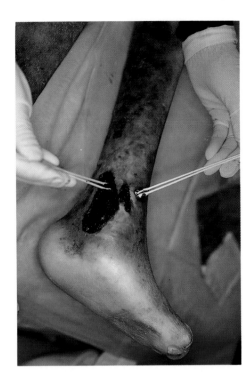

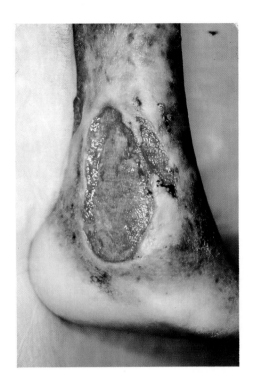

Figure 10.2a
Zinc chloride paste debridement

The black colored, zinc chloride paste as used in the original Mohs micrographic technique is an effective debriding agent. The thickness of paste applied will determine the depth of debridement. The procedure produces moderate discomfort.

Figure 10.2b
Zinc chloride paste debridement/Follow up

One week after the application of zinc chloride, the black paste and necrotic tissue sloughed off spontaneously. As originally noted by Dr. Mohs, the granulation tissue appears healthier than would be predicted.

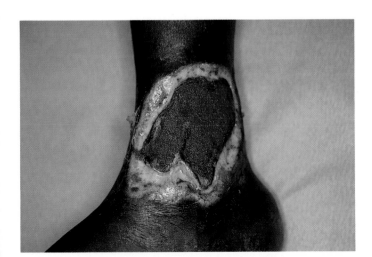

Figure 10.3a
Zinc chloride paste debridement

This sickle cell ulcer had suffered from repeated bouts of infection with Pseudomonas. Treatment with zinc chloride was used to debride the ulcer. Most of the base contains a black eschar induced by the zinc chloride treatment.

Continued

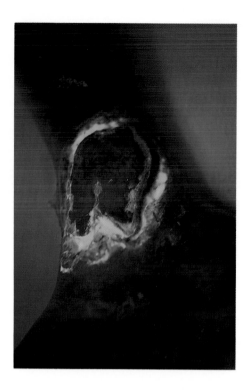

Figure 10.3b
Zinc chloride paste debridement/Wood's light

The edges fluoresce greenish-yellow indicating tissue invasion by Pseudomonas. Wood's light examination offers a quick diagnosis of Pseudomonas infection.

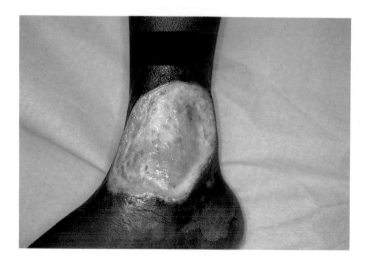

Figure 10.3c
Zinc chloride paste debridement/ Follow up

The eschar formed by zinc chloride paste came off spontaneously leaving a faintly pink base. The infection has not fully resolved as suggested by the yellowish exudate at the edges and in the upper portion of the ulcer bed. This patient's ulcer might be treated with a second application of zinc chloride paste.

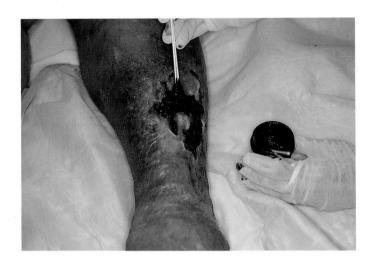

Figure 10.4a
Zinc chloride paste debridement

The black zinc chloride paste is being applied to the ulcer base with a cotton applicator. Zinc chloride does not penetrate intact skin but it is still wise to protect the surrounding skin with petrolatum.

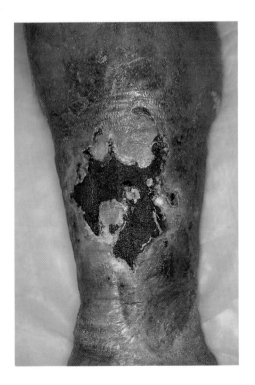

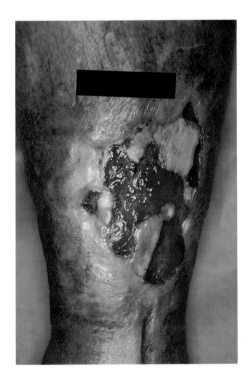

Figure 10.4b
Zinc chloride paste debridement/Several days after application

Figure 10.4c
Zinc chloride paste debridement/Follow up

The eschar has sloughed off after several days, leaving good granulation tissue.

Continued

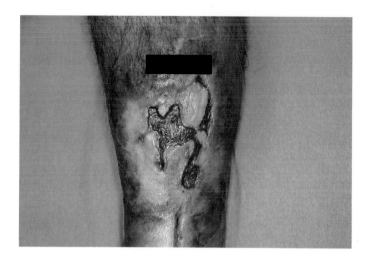

Figure 10.4d
**Zinc chloride paste debridement/
Follow up**

Six weeks later, the ulcer is considerably smaller and continues to have a healthy looking granulation tissue base.

11 Exudation

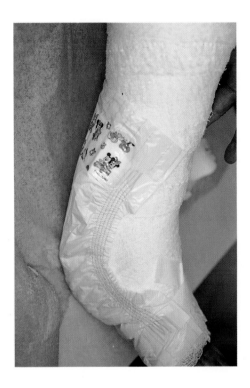

Figure 11.1
Baby diaper to control exudate

A diaper is applied over the wound dressing and the gauze to absorb the exudate until the Unna boot is changed next week. The diaper is wrapped in with another layer of gauze. We have found that diaper application around the ulcer benefits a few patients with excessive exudate. Although this method to control exudate may seem facetious, it does point out the effectiveness of this type of material and the opportunity to develop more feasible absorbent dressings.

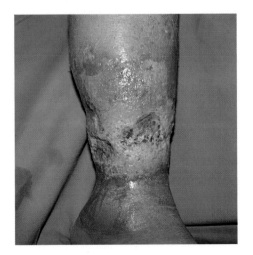

Figure 11.2
Edematous, weeping, ulcerated leg

These patients need acute hospital care. Antibiotics should be given intravenously.

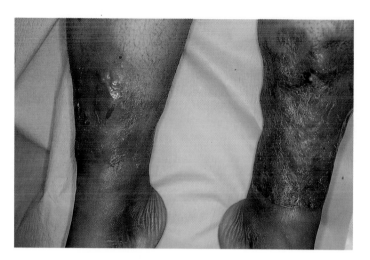

Figure 11.3
Recurrent abscesses

In this ulcer diagnosed as pyoderma gangrenosum, cultures taken from the ulcer tissue grew *Mycobacterium chelonei*. The patient then improved with antibiotic therapy. Her skin has become hyperpigmented and nodular and there are many draining sinuses.

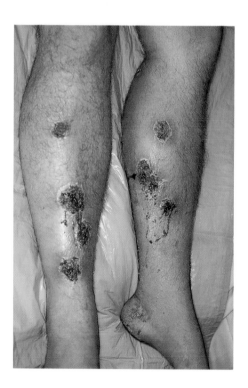

Figure 11.4a
Pyoderma

These crusted lesions were initially very exudative. They were due to streptococcal infection. The red borders are quite characteristic.

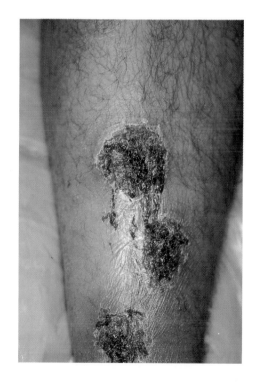

Figure 11.4b
Pyoderma/Close-up

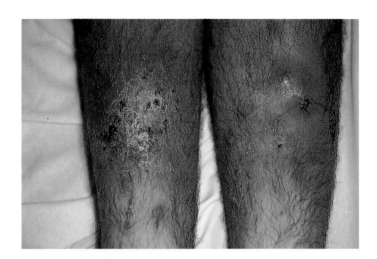

Figure 11.5a
Acne fulminans

The abscesses and highly exudative pretibial lesions in this 17-year-old boy were a diagnostic dilemma for some time. Biopsies did not show evidence of vasculitis or infection. His presentation included constitutional symptoms, anemia and bone lytic lesions.

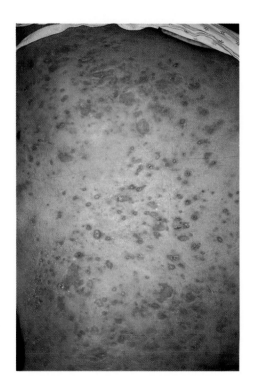

Figure 11.5b
Acne fulminans/Diagnosis

His back and chest were covered by an acneiform eruption, which had developed at the same time as the leg lesions. He had been practicing muscle building but denied taking androgenic steroids. Treatment with systemic corticosteroids produced a dramatic improvement in his condition.

12 Granulation tissue

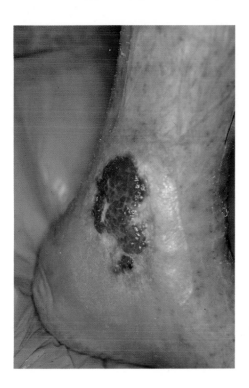

Figure 12.1
Overgrown granulation tissue

The skin around the excessive granulation tissue is hydrated because an occlusive dressing had recently been removed. We treat this overgrowth of granulation tissue by discontinuing the use of occlusive dressings.

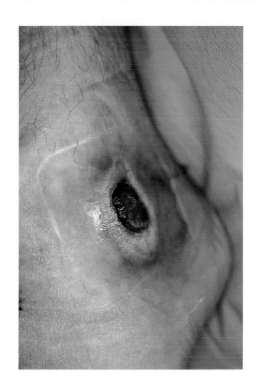

Figure 12.2
Neuropathic ulcer in a paraplegic

A hydrocolloid dressing has just been removed. The granulation tissue in ulcers beneath hydrocolloid dressings is often beefy and dusky. Within hours the tissues become a lighter red color.

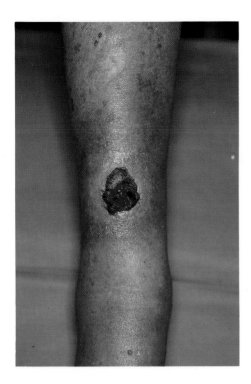

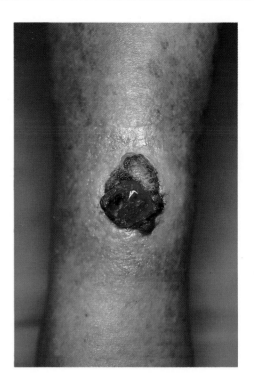

Figure 12.3a
Exophytic ulcer of the ankle

Figure 12.3b
Exophytic ulcer of the ankle/Close-up

This lady had a pre-leukemic state including thrombocytopenia. Following mild household trauma to her leg, an exophytic ulcerative lesion developed at the site of injury. An excisional biopsy showed histologic evidence of pyogenic granuloma. The lesion did not heal and in fact enlarged until the patient died a few months later.

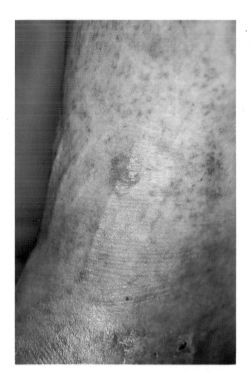

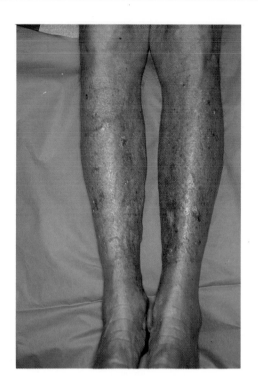

Figure 12.4
Basal cell carcinoma on the leg

The photograph shows a basal cell carcinoma overlying a superficial vein. It has often been speculated that basal cell carcinomas are more common in venous disease.

Figure 12.5
Multiple basal cell carcinomas

Multiple basal cell carcinomas in an elderly man with severe actinic damage and venous disease. They may initially appear to be multiple ulcers with good granulation tissue.

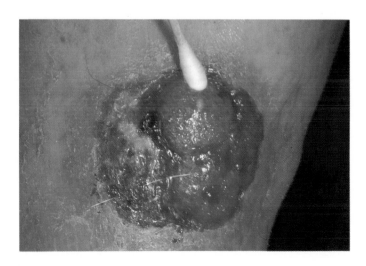

Figure 12.6
Basal cell carcinoma in a venous ulcer

This exophytic mass was misdiagnosed as exuberant granulation tissue for more than a year. Compression treatment reduced the size of the mass and allowed partial reepithelialization. Partial reepithelialization with episodes of regression should be another clue to the possibility of basal cell carcinoma.

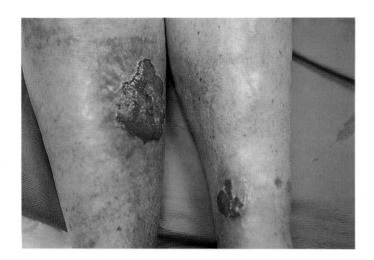

Figure 12.7
Basal cell carcinoma mimicking healthy granulation tissue

This 76-year-old woman had non-healing leg ulcers for more than two years. The raised and lobulated appearance of the "granulation tissue" led us to biopsy the ulcer bed. As expected, the histology showed basal cell carcinomas in both ulcers.

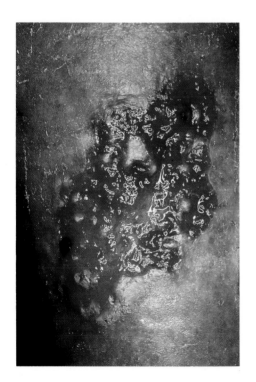

Figure 12.8
Basal cell carcinoma in a venous ulcer

This is another example of basal cell carcinoma resembling good granulation tissue. Biopsy of the ulcer bed confirmed the diagnosis of basal cell carcinoma. The lobulated and "glassy" appearance of the "granulation tissue" which seems to roll over to cover the surrounding skin is a good clue to the presence of this malignancy. One should not be led astray by the apparent areas of reepithelialization which can be seen throughout the tumor.

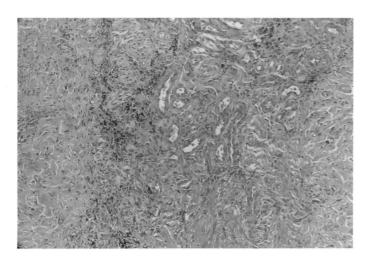

Figure 12.9
Venous ulcer histology

The thickened and tortuous superficial vessel can be appreciated in
this field as can the dermal pigment
in the melanophages. The biopsy
was from the wound bed of a non-
healing venous ulcer.

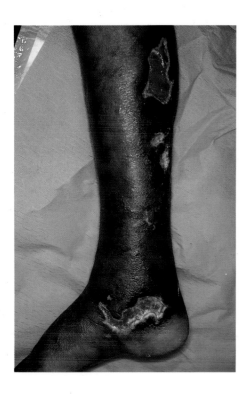

Figure 12.10
***Vibrio vulnificus* infection**

The granulation tissue in these acute leg ulcers
is quite good. The ulcers are due to a systemic
infection with *Vibrio vulnificus*, which the
patient contracted after pricking his hand with a
fishing hook while fishing off the Florida coast.
Infection with Vibrio is particularly common in
patients with hemochromatosis (as in this man)
or other iron overload states.

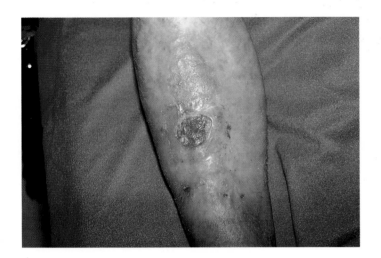

Figure 12.11
Factitial ulcer

The granulation tissue in this elderly retarded man's ulcer is quite good, but the ulcer did not epithelialize. He had good arterial blood flow and no evidence of venous disease. There was no clear explanation for the ulcer. His nurses finally observed him scraping the ulcer with a pocket knife. Protection of the ulcer with an Unna boot led to complete healing within four weeks.

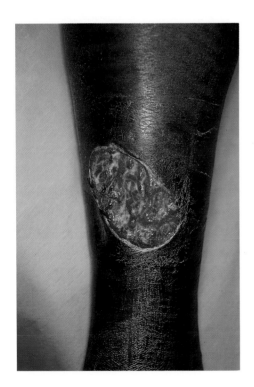

Figure 12.12
Unusual ulcer in a patient with AIDS

At first, the ulcer bed might appear to represent granulation tissue. However, the duration of the ulcer (several months) and the substantial ulcer depth caused us to suspect an unusual process. The male patient did not have findings consistent with common etiologies, including venous disease, arterial insufficiency and sickle cell hemoglobinopathy. A biopsy and culture of the tissue showed infection with *Mycobacterium chelonei*. A high degree of suspicion must be present when evaluating ulcers in immuno-compromised patients.

13 Necrosis

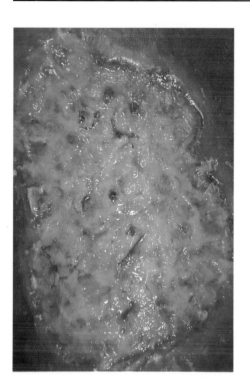

Figure 13.1
Venous ulcer with gelatinous necrosis

The linear and punctate gray areas in the upper and central portion of this ulcer are necrotic blood vessels, as demonstrated histologically. Cuts made with a scalpel in the lower portion of the ulcer show healthy looking granulation tissue underneath the surface dermal necrosis. It is often possible to debride such ulcers almost painlessly. We have seen gelatinous necrosis appear during sudden worsening of the ulcer and, rarely, under occlusive dressings. Gelatinous necrosis appears to represent denatured collagen and other tissue macromolecules.

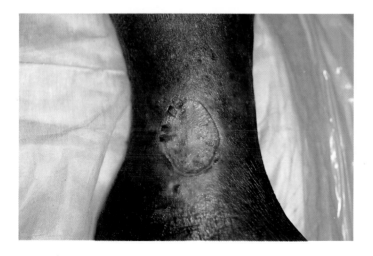

Figure 13.2
Venous ulcer with four biopsy sites

This is an excellent example of an ulcer with gelatinous necrosis. The reasonably large biopsies do not bleed excessively and heal up to the pre-existing ulcer edge without difficulty. Sutures are not used. The biopsies encompass and allow examination of both the wound bed and the adjacent non-ulcerated skin.

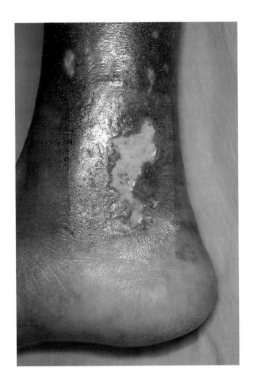

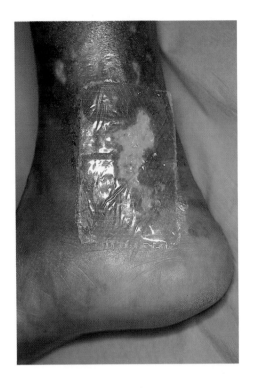

Figure 13.3a
Ulcer in a sickle cell anemia patient

This is another excellent example of gelatinous necrosis, which is a common occurrence in this type of ulceration. These ulcers tend to be particularly painful.

Figure 13.3b
**Ulcer in a sickle cell anemia patient/
Treatment**

We often use occlusive dressings to achieve painless debridement. A gel dressing was used in this case because of its superior capacity to ease pain.

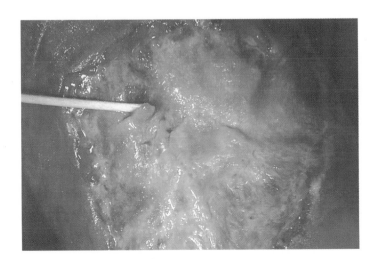

Figure 13.4
Gelatinous necrosis

As illustrated, the necrotic material can be peeled off with a cotton applicator. Healthy appearing granulation tissue is found below the necrotic material.

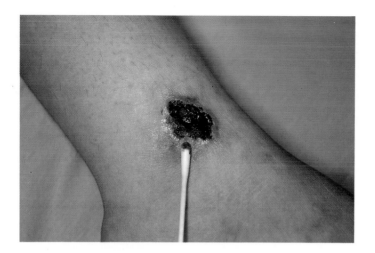

Figure 13.5
Ulcer with factitial necrosis

Although it appeared that the surface of this ulcer had become necrotic, the color was in fact secondary to applications of herbal remedies and it could be scraped away.

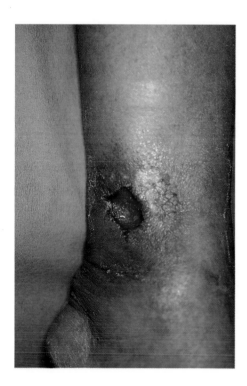

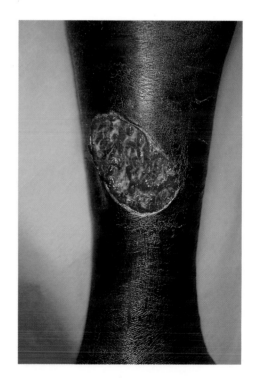

Figure 13.6
Venous ulcer — unusually painful

We have several patients with established venous disease whose ulcers are in the usual site for venous ulceration but are unusually small, deep and painful.

Figure 13.7
Infectious ulcer — *Mycobacterium chelonei*

This ulcer was on the lateral side of the leg and the extent of necrosis is more than one would expect in venous disease. There were no signs of arterial disease and no hemoglobinopathy. A biopsy was sent for culture. The patient was later found to be HIV positive.

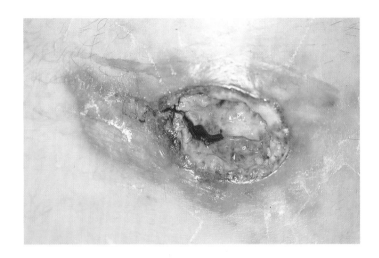

Figure 13.8
Ulcer — lymphoma

This ulcer had been diagnosed as pyoderma gangrenosum. We took many biopsies from within the ulcer and from its edge. Only after a large biopsy which extended from the ulcer edge well into the adjacent skin, was the diagnosis of lymphoma made. A complete work-up led to the diagnosis of systemic B-cell lymphoma. This illustrates the importance of taking biopsies extending well beyond the ulcer edge.

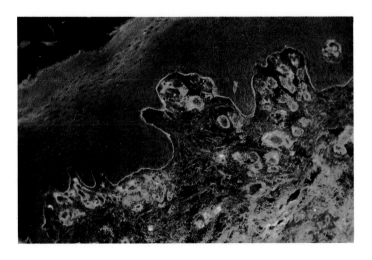

Figure 13.9
Necrotic foot ulcer in systemic sclerosis

This 67-year-old woman with systemic sclerosis developed this ulceration quite suddenly. There was no evidence of vascular thrombosis or the antiphospholipid syndrome. Autoamputation was the eventual outcome, and no surgical procedures were necessary.

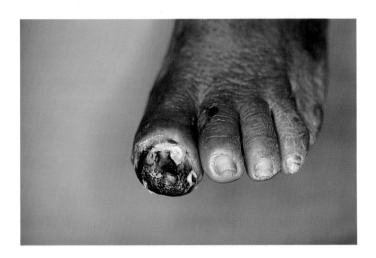

Figure 13.10a
Pericapillary fibrin cuffs

One hypothesis for venous ulceration suggests that venous hypertension leads to dermal leakage of fibrinogen and pericapillary fibrin cuffs, which prevent the diffusion of oxygen and other nutrients. This photograph illustrates these fibrin cuffs in tissue taken from a venous ulcer bed. The tissue sections were stained with an antibody to fibrinogen/fibrin and examined by direct immunofluorescence.

Continued

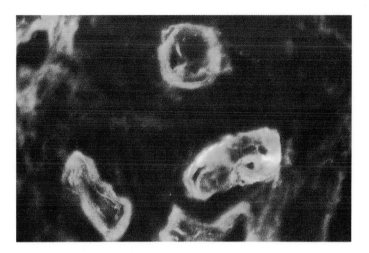

Figure 13.10b
Pericapillary fibrin cuffs/Close-up

Fibrin cuffs are present in most venous ulcers and lipodermato-sclerotic tissue, although they are not totally specific for venous disease. A more recent hypothesis for the pathogenesis of venous ulceration (the "trap" hypothesis) suggests that in addition to vascular leakage of fibrinogen there is extra-vasation of other macromolecules, including alpha-2-macroglobulin. The extravasated macromolecules bind or "trap" growth factors and normal matrix material and make them unavailable for ulcer healing and tissue integrity.

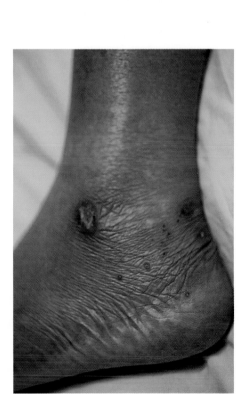

Figure 13.11
Herpetic ulcers

These necrotic foot ulcers were painless but persistent in this immunocompromised man with a kidney transplant. Biopsy and Tzanck smear both showed multinucleated giant cells, and cultures grew Herpes simplex. These embolic lesions are probably the result of viremia.

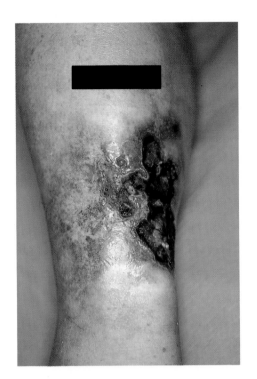

Figure 13.12a
Cryoglobulinemia

Necrosis and necrotic tissue within the ulcer bed is extremely rare in venous disease. The photograph also illustrates redness and atrophy surrounding the ulceration. This female patient had cryoglobulinemia.

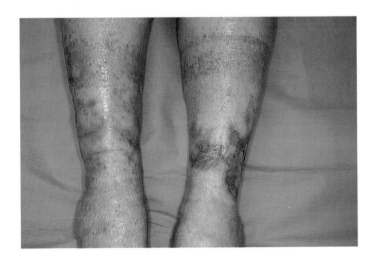

Figure 13.12b
Cryoglobulinemia/Follow up

Treatment with intravenous pulse corticosteroids and azathioprine healed the ulcer.

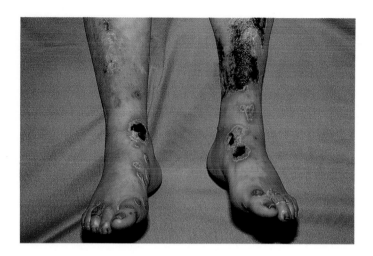

Figure 13.13
Leukocytoclastic vasculitis

These necrotic lesions developed after this elderly man took thiazide diuretics for treatment of his hypertension. Histology showed leukocytoclastic vasculitis.

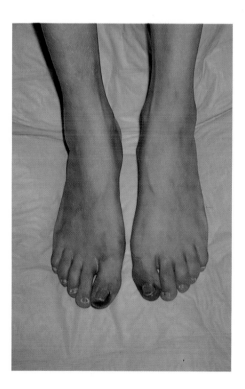

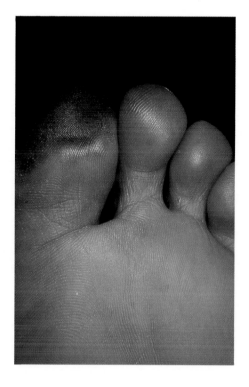

Figure 13.14a
Antiphospholipid syndrome

This young woman with systemic lupus erythematosus developed gangrenous lesions on her toes. The involved area on the right foot was outlined with ink to better follow the progression of the lesion. Work-up revealed the presence of a lupus anticoagulant.

Figure 13.14b
Antiphospholipid syndrome/Close-up

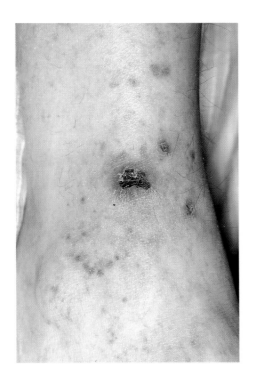

Figure 13.15a
Cholesterol embolization

This middle aged man developed purpuric lesions and a necrotic ulcer. He also had constitutional symptoms and renal failure. Peripheral pulses were quite adequate, a finding that is characteristic of cholesterol embolization. There was no recent history of vascular surgery or vascular radiographic procedures.

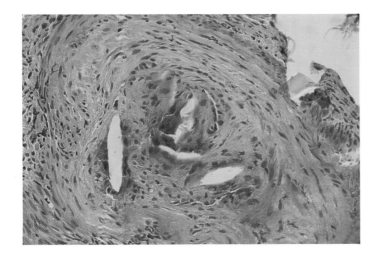

Figure 13.15b
Cholesterol embolization/ Histology

Histological examination of biopsy material taken from the ulcer showed the typical "cholesterol clefts" that are diagnostic for this life-threatening condition. Frequently, serial sections of biopsy material are necessary to establish the diagnosis.

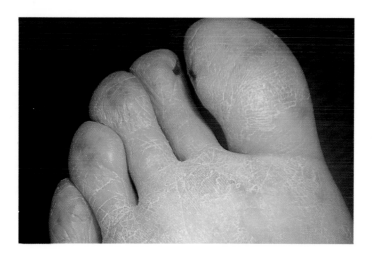

Figure 13.16a
Cholesterol emboli

In this other man with cholesterol embolization, several typical skin findings were present. Here one sees the purple discoloration of the toes that is common in this disease.

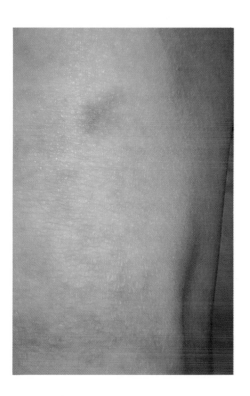

Figure 13.16b
Cholesterol emboli/Livedo

Livedo reticularis is the most common skin finding in patients with cholesterol embolization. As was the case here, livedo lesions are frequently present on the thighs and may extend to the trunk.

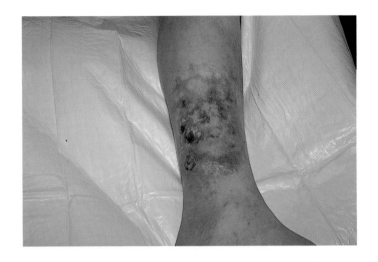

Figure 13.17
Cryofibrinogenemia

As is often the case with ulcers due to this undiagnosed condition, this female patient had been treated with repeated courses of systemic antibiotics without improvement. The presence of necrotic ulcers and the livedo pattern observed superiorly are typical of this entity.

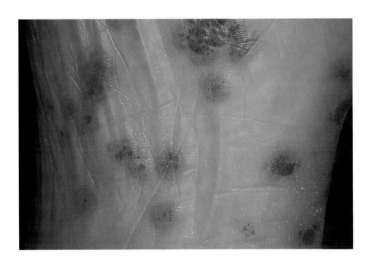

Figure 13.18
Septic emboli

These sole lesions were present in a man with bacterial endocarditis. The location, necrosis and hemorrhage surrounded by a red halo were highly suggestive of a septic process. It is uncommon for these lesions to ulcerate.

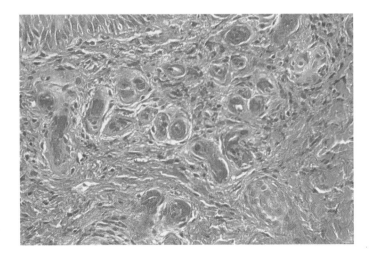

Figure 13.19
Intravascular fibrin thrombi

This histological picture is seen in disseminated intravascular coagulation, thrombotic thrombocytopenic purpura, cryoglobulinemia, cryofibrinogenemia, and thrombosis of larger "upstream" blood vessels. The antiphospholipid syndrome is characterized also by a rather marked perivascular inflammatory process, which is not seen here.

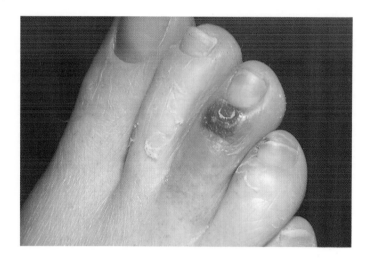

Figure 13.20
Aspergillosis

This 38-year-old man had recently received multiple organ transplants and was on immunosuppressive therapy. The necrotic center of this toe lesion with surrounding redness is frequently seen in infections due to Aspergillus. Biopsy confirmed this. Other lesions were present on the patient's legs, face and trunk. He responded well to systemic antifungal therapy.

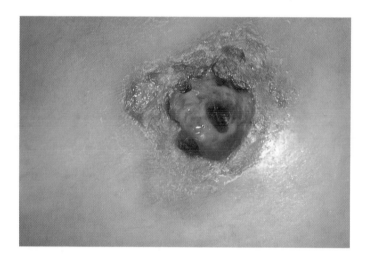

Figure 13.21
Lymphoma

For several months, this calf ulcer with deep necrosis and undermined edges in a young woman was thought to be pyoderma gangrenosum. However, high doses of systemic corticosteroids failed to improve it. We repeated a wedge biopsy from the edge of the ulcer, but the histology was non-specific. Not satisfied, we then performed another, larger biopsy extending about three centimeters from the edge into seemingly normal skin. Histological examination of this tissue showed a histiocytic lymphoma. Further work-up then revealed abdominal lymph node involvement.

Clinical points

- Calcification is very common in venous disease and ulceration.
- Zinc chloride paste is a very effective but somewhat painful method of ulcer debridement.
- The edges of ulcers treated with occlusive dressings will be hydrated and appear white upon dressing removal.
- Occlusion promotes the formation of granulation tissue and occasionally causes it to become very exuberant.
- Basal cell carcinoma within ulcers looks like overgrown granulation tissue.
- Typically, biopsies of venous ulcers heal up to the pre-existing ulcer edge.
- If a malignancy (such as lymphoma) is suspected as the cause of the ulceration, biopsies should extend well beyond the ulcer's edge.
- Patients with cholesterol embolization often have a recent history of vascular surgery or vascular radiographic procedures.
- Livedo reticularis is the most common skin finding in patients with cholesterol embolization.

IV   EPITHELIUM

Introduction

Failure to heal is the hallmark of chronic leg ulcers. In the preceding sections we have emphasized the diagnostic features of many types of leg ulcers and an approach to their management. The next two sections are concerned more with the inability of the epidermis to either develop or persist within the ulcers. Perhaps no ulcer poses this dilemma with better clarity than the venous ulcer. It is perplexing that venous ulcers will often not re-epithelialize in spite of seemingly optimal granulation tissue. In fact, there is increasing evidence that the hypertrophic epidermis at the edges of venous ulcers is in an "activated" state of increased expression of growth factor receptors and other cytokines. Occasionally, however, failure of leg ulcers to heal is the result of extrinsic factors. We have emphasized several of these factors in this section.

A relatively common problem is the use of antiseptics and other topical agents that delay healing. We prefer to use only saline in ulcerated tissue. Another common problem occurs during the course of therapy with occlusive dressings. At the start of therapy with adherent occlusive dressings, such as films and hydrocolloids, patients are forced to change dressings because of the exudate. As the ulcer heals and less exudate is produced, the correct way is to leave the dressings on for as long as possible. However, manufacturers' indications and, often, the advice of health care workers to patients is to change dressings at set intervals. What then happens is that the newly formed epidermis in an ulcer that is no longer exudative is often stripped during dressing removal. Once this problem is identified, the easiest approach is to discontinue adhesive occlusive dressings altogether. Recognition of this problem is not always easy. However, as described in this section, we have found that newly resurfaced areas of ulcers are often detected by wrinkling the transparent epithelium with a cotton applicator.

Ulcers which contain apparently healthy granulation tissue but which do not re-epithelialize should be treated with partial thickness skin grafts. In addition to replacing tissue, grafts have a pharmacologic effect that provides a stimulus to the wound bed and to the ulcer edge.

14 Failure of reepithelialization

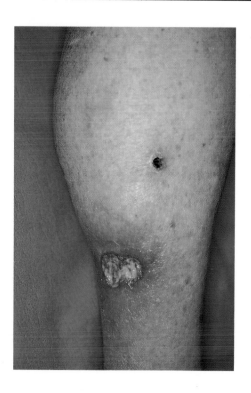

Figure 14.1
Squamous cell carcinoma arising in a leg that was irradiated 55 years earlier

After the carcinoma was removed, the resulting ulceration did not heal. This is an example of the long latency period between x-irradiation and neoplasia. The patient also illustrates the difficulty in healing skin that has been previously x-irradiated.

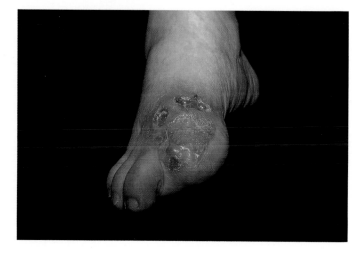

Figure 14.2
Factitial ulceration

This 66-year-old woman even convinced her physicians that her ulcerations were due to a specific disease process. She underwent removal of the entire big toe and many grafting procedures. She did not have arterial disease and also had no evidence of vasculitis on biopsy and no laboratory evidence of cryoglobulinemia. Therapy with an Unna boot to prevent her from manipulating her ulceration produced substantial improvement before she was "lost to follow up".

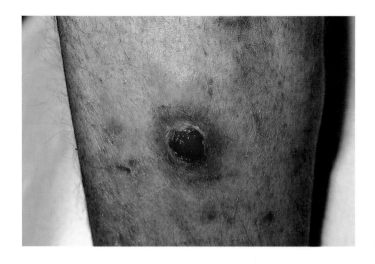

Figure 14.3
Basal cell carcinoma arising from a venous ulcer

Islands of epithelium arising from the edge of this lesion could make the diagnosis of basal cell carcinoma difficult clinically. However, the lobulated granulation-type appearance of the wound bed should make one suspicious that this is a basal cell carcinoma.

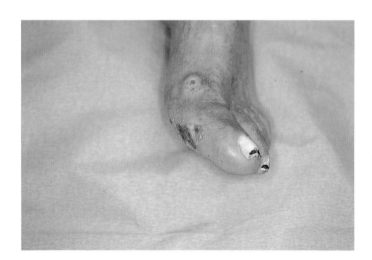

Figure 14.4a
Invasive dermatophyte infection

This man was not immunocompromised but had a long history of a dermatophyte infection of his feet which was unresponsive to conventional systemic treatment. He was referred after he developed an ulcer in his metatarsal area that failed to heal with hydrocolloid dressing therapy.

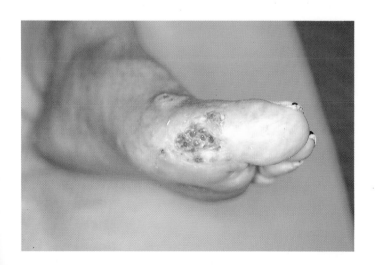

Figure 14.4b
Invasive dermatophyte infection/ Close up

There is a remnant of hydrocolloid on the superior distal edge. On histological examination of the wound bed there were fungal elements deep in dermis. Culture of the wound biopsy material showed evidence of infection with *T. rubrum*. He responded and the ulcer healed after several series of hospital treatments with intravenous amphotericin.

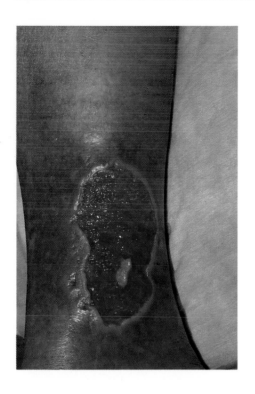

Figure 14.5

Island of epithelial tissue in a venous ulcer

The ulcer bed is made of healthy appearing granulation tissue. Nevertheless, epidermal migration does not occur from the edges or from the island of epithelium. This preserved island of intact skin is a tremendous biological puzzle. How it survives where epithelium will not migrate is unknown.

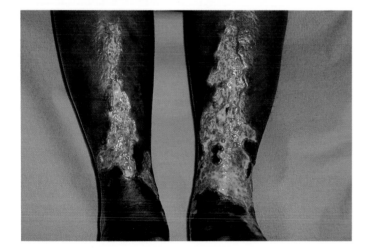

Figure 14.6

"Rebound" from stanozolol therapy

This patient initially had small ulcerations. She had cryofibrinogenemia and small vessel thrombi on biopsy of the ulcers. She was started on 4 mg a day of stanozolol and, after about three weeks, the ulcers were improving. However, we were forced to stop stanozolol abruptly because of rising liver enzymes. Within a week, her ulcers markedly increased in size and new ones developed on both legs (as shown here). This case and others we have observed have convinced us that, if at all possible, one should taper stanozolol therapy slowly.

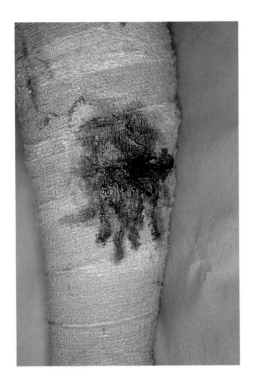

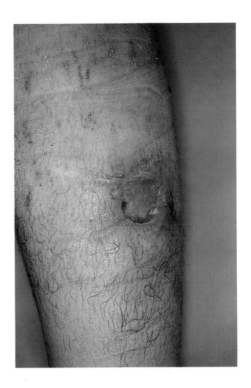

Figure 14.7a
Factitial ulceration

This 23-year-old girl had an ulcer on her calf
and gave a history of healing problems after
trauma or surgical excision. Her family history
was negative for similar problems and she did
not have over-stretchable skin or over-
extensible joints. Because we suspected the ulcer
was self induced, an Unna paste boot followed
by a self adherent wrap was placed over the leg.
When seen in one week, the linear blood stains
again suggested manipulation by the patient.

Figure 14.7b
**Factitial ulceration/Immediately after
removing the Unna boot**

The indentations left by the compression
bandage can still be seen. The ulcer appears
healthy. Fresh and crusted scratch marks distant
from the ulcer can be seen. Many of these are at
the upper border of the Unna boot, an area she
might have been able to reach more easily.

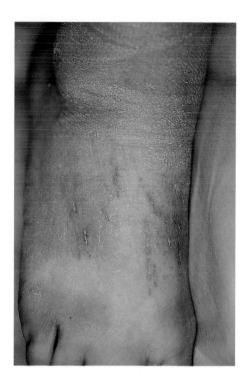

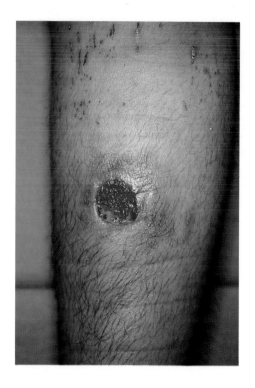

Figure 14.7c
Factitial ulceration/Signs

Similar linear excoriations can be seen at the anterior border of the foot area that was covered by the Unna boot.

Figure 14.7d
Factitial ulceration/Follow up

Treatment with the Unna boot protection was continued. After three weeks of treatment the ulcer was filled with beefy red granulation tissue.

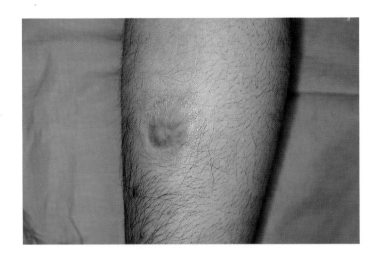

Figure 14.7e
Factitial ulceration/Protective therapy

After six weeks of protection by Unna boot the ulcer has completely healed.

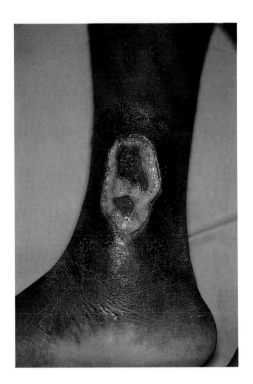

Figure 14.8
Ulcer due to sickle cell anemia

This is an excellent example of yellow gelatinous necrosis that is often recurrent in some ulcers. It may occur suddenly, and sometimes after the use of occlusive dressings. As seen in other situations, two non-ulcerated areas have become islands of skin within the ulcer. Interestingly, reepithelialization does not occur from these islands. Ulcers in sickle cell anemia are often deeper and more painful than venous ulcers.

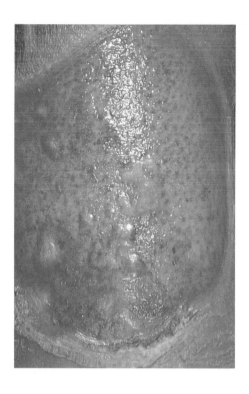

Figure 14.9
Reepithelialization of a venous ulcer

Epithelium can be seen at the edges and also from within the center of the ulcer. It is very unusual to see central reepithelialization in ulcers of this depth.

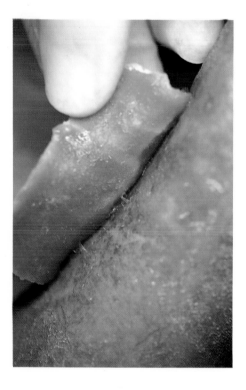

Figure 14.10
Epithelial stripping by an occlusive dressing

This photograph illustrates the ability of an occlusive dressing to "strip" stratum corneum and epithelium from the skin adjacent to an ulcer. Appreciating this potential, we either extend the wearing time or discontinue occlusive dressings if an ulcer that appears to have responded favorably to occlusive dressings does not totally reepithelialize.

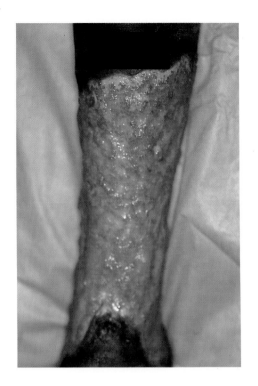

Figure 14.11
Sickle cell ulcer

A large circumferential ulcer in a woman with hemoglobin C. In this case, the granulation tissue appears adequate, but the epithelium does not migrate over this wound bed. The etiologies of leg ulceration in patients with hemoglobino-pathies have not been studied in detail. These ulcers appear to have both a venous and an arteriolar component.

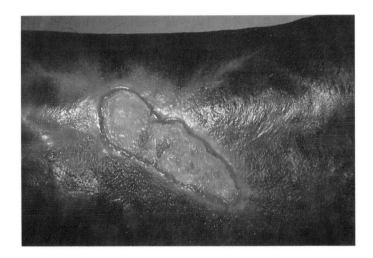

Figure 14.12
Ulcer due to sickle cell anemia

This man's ulcer was, typically, quite painful. The ulcer was larger, and the hypopigmented skin around it indicates areas that have recently reepithelialized. However, no evidence of epidermal resurfacing is present at this time.

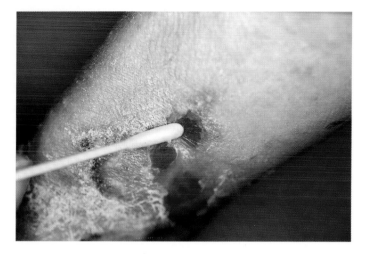

Figure 14.13
"Wrinkle test" for epidermal resurfacing

It is quite obvious that these ulcers have excellent granulation tissue, but the thin epithelial layer that covers them is not readily apparent. This photograph illustrates a simple procedure, the "wrinkle test". A cotton applicator gently pressed at an angle to the surface of the ulcer demonstrates multiple fine wrinkles that represent a thin epidermal layer. The test is helpful when following ulcers that fail to heal with adherent occlusive dressings, since this thin epidermal layer suggests that dressings are causing repeated trauma to the reepithelialization process and should be discontinued.

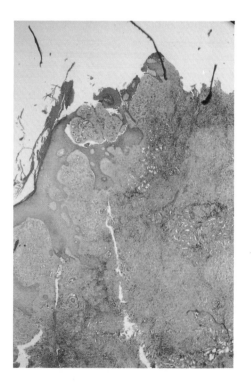

Figure 14.14
Edge of venous ulcer

The hyperplastic and hyperproliferative epidermis observed in this photomicrograph is typical. Failure of this epidermis to migrate across the wound is a biologic puzzle.

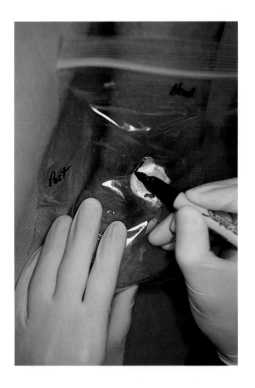

Figure 14.15a
Ulcer size measurements

Occlusive film dressings have been developed that will allow the clinician to keep track of the extent of reepithelialization during treatment. Other more sophisticated techniques are also available. For the last several years, we have made use of a simple double sided "sandwich bag" to keep a permanent record of ulcer measurements. The bag is placed over the ulcer and a felt tip pen is used to outline the ulcer's perimeter. The water vapor that forms immediately after occlusion of the ulcer is often useful in establishing the outline.

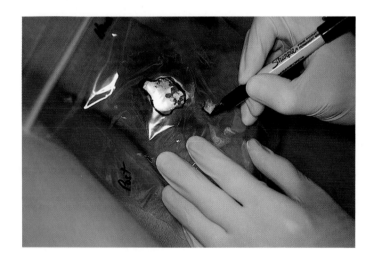

Figure 14.15b
**Ulcer size measurements/
Continued**

Multiple ulcers can be outlined this way on the same piece of plastic.

Continued

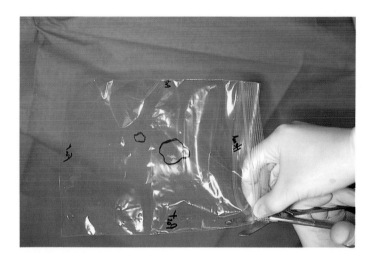

Figure 14.15c
**Ulcer size measurements/
Continued**

Using scissors, the side of the bag
that was in contact with the ulcer
can be cut away and discarded.

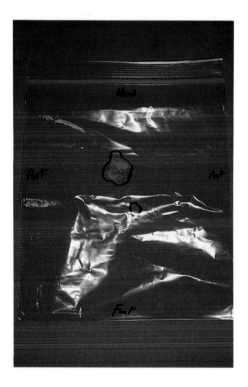

Figure 14.15d
Ulcer size measurements/Continued

This leaves a plastic sheet with a permanent
record of the size of the ulcers.

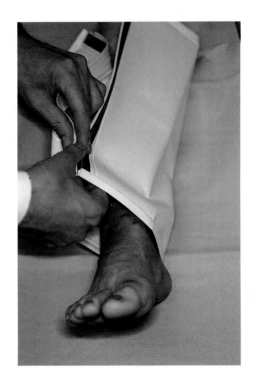

Figure 14.16
Air plethysmography

Whenever ulcers fail to heal, their etiology must be reconsidered. Here, one of our patients with a presumed venous leg ulcer is being tested for the presence of venous disease by air plethysmography. This special sensing cuff will be filled with air up to a selectable pressure and several measurements will be made, including venous filling and ejection index.

15 Grafts

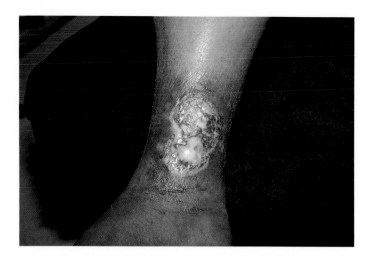

Figure 15.1
Graft with pus-filled blister

Pus-filled blisters occurred in this
non-meshed, partial-thickness graft
after two weeks. Some portions of
the graft took but much needed to
be cut away. Meshed grafts allow
wound fluid to escape from the ulcer
and these are our preferred method
of grafting.

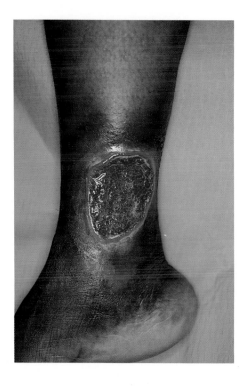

Figure 15.2a
Venous ulcer

A healthy granulation bed can develop but the
epithelial edges of the ulcer do not migrate.
Grafting will shorten the healing time.

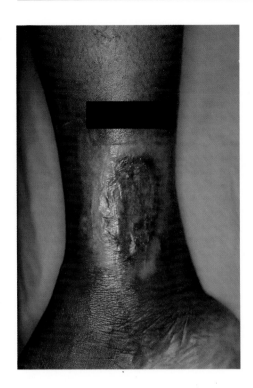

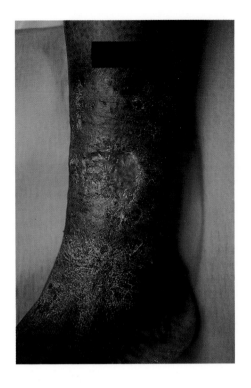

Figure 15.2b
Venous ulcer/After grafting

Graded compression stockings must be worn to prevent recurrence. Most venous ulcers can be healed, but recurrences are difficult to prevent. Recurrences occur within the grafted site and elsewhere in the gaiter area.

Figure 15.3a
Non-healing venous ulcer

The ulcer bed is lifeless and there is no healing from the edge.

Continued

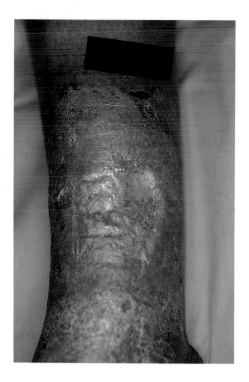

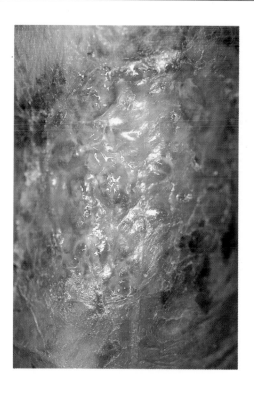

Figure 15.3b
Non-healing venous ulcer/After out-patient pinch grafting

The ulcer bed looks healthier with islands of granulation tissue. Pinch grafts were applied in the ambulatory setting every three days to obtain this pharmacologic rather than tissue replacement effect.

Figure 15.4
Ulcer recurrence shortly after successful grafting

Three weeks after successful grafting, wet and yellow-appearing holes occurred in some parts of the graft. At some sites the holes have an extrusion of red granulation-like tissue.

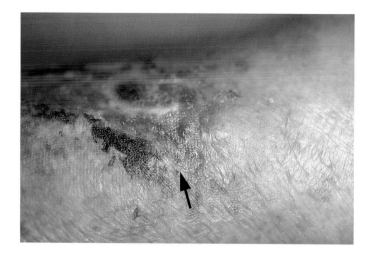

Figure 15.5
Grafted ulcer

The new epithelium can be seen migrating from the hydrated edge of the pinch graft near the center of this ulcer. A similar pink sheet of epithelium can be seen extending from the edge toward the graft (arrow). The original border of the ulcer's edge is marked with black ink.

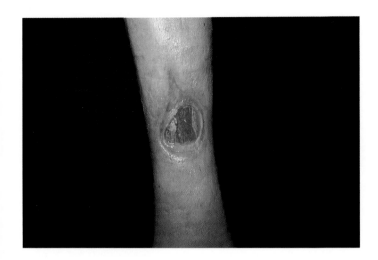

Figure 15.6a
Ulcerated surgical scar

This elderly woman developed an ulcer in a surgical scar after an operation for arterial revascularization. Bone, tendon and fat can be seen in the base of this ulcer on the medial aspect of her shin.

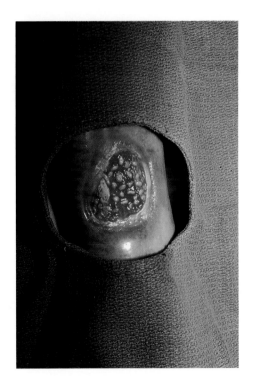

Figure 15.6b
Ulcerated surgical scar/Immediately following pinch grafting

Because her ulcer would not heal and the limb had already been revascularized, we chose to treat her with pinch grafts for their pharmacologic effect.

Continued

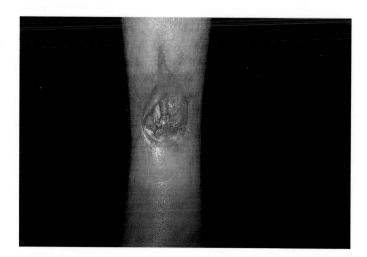

Figure 15.6c
Ulcerated surgical scar/Healed

Following pinch grafting, the ulcer healed. The spicule of bone seen in the bed of a portion of this ulcer confounded us for awhile. Ultimately, this spicule was removed for us by a surgical colleague who found the ulcer was totally reepithelialized below the bony spicule.

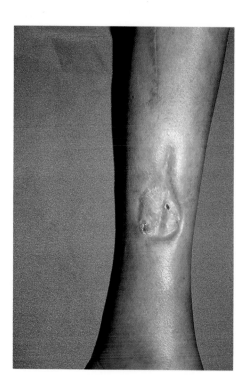

Figure 15.6d
Ulcerated surgical scar/Follow up

The site remained healed after several months of observation.

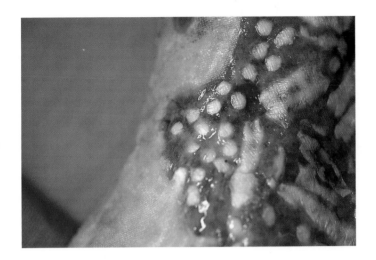

Figure 15.7
Split-thickness grafts — different sizes and shapes

Occasionally, we still use pinch grafts for treatment of leg ulcers, especially if a pharmacologic effect is being sought. As illustrated in this photograph, there is no need to limit the shape and sizes of these grafts: small pinch grafts can be used side by side with thin long strips of donor skin.

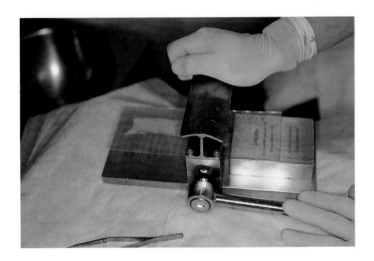

Figure 15.8
Meshed grafts

A sheet of split-thickness donor skin is being meshed so that it may cover a large leg ulcer and allow wound fluid to escape from the grafted site.

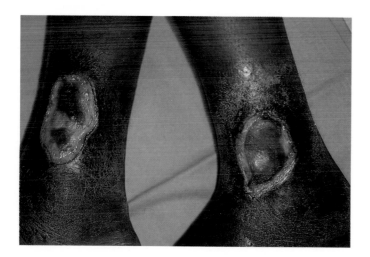

Figure 15.9
Failed grafts in sickle cell anemia ulcers

We have had disappointing results in grafting ulcers in patients with sickle cell anemia. This photograph shows the failed "shrunken" grafts three weeks after the procedure in a patient in his early 30s.

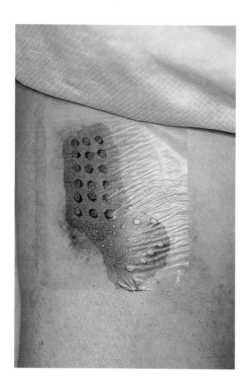

Figure 15.10
Graft donor site treated with occlusion

A film dressing was used to treat these thigh wounds from which punch biopsy grafts had been harvested. Occlusive dressings ease the pain and speed up the process of reepithelialization in this type of wound. This "acute" wound fluid developed beneath the dressing after 24 hours and could be aspirated without removing the dressing. The same type of wound fluid has been shown to promote the growth of endothelial cells and fibroblasts, while "chronic" wound fluid from venous ulcers inhibits the in vitro proliferation of keratinocytes, endothelial cells and fibroblasts.

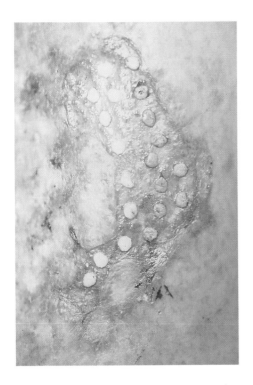

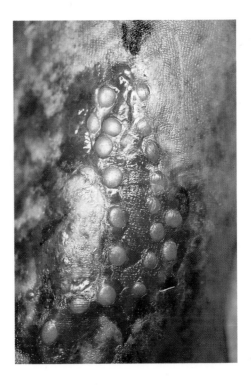

Figure 15.11a
Grafts as pharmacologic agents

The subcutaneous tissue and fat were removed from donor "punch grafts" and the grafts were then applied to this ulcer to stimulate the formation of granulation tissue and reepithelialization.

Figure 15.11b
Grafts as pharmacologic agents/Follow up

A few days later a remarkable improvement in the granulation tissue has been obtained. All the grafts appear viable. We often place grafts repeatedly (every few days or weeks) to stimulate ulcer healing.

Clinical points

- Good granulation tissue does not always lead to epithelialization, nor does epithelialization always depend upon good granulation tissue.
- Venous ulcers are often characterized by failure of epithelialization in spite of good granulation tissue.
- The application of an Unna boot is a good way to deal with factitial leg ulcerations.
- Yellow gelatinous necrosis may occur after the use of occlusive dressings.
- Adherent occlusive dressings may strip stratum corneum and healthy epithelium in the late, non-exudative phases of ulcer healing.
- Newly formed, transparent epidermis is often missed. It can be "wrinkled" and becomes more apparent upon touching its surface with a cotton applicator.
- Meshed grafts are preferred in the treatment of leg ulcers because they allow wound fluid to escape rather than lift off the graft.
- Graded compression stockings must be worn to prevent recurrence of venous ulcers.
- Grafts applied to ulcers stimulate granulation tissue and epidermal resurfacing from the ulcer's edge. This may be considered a pharmacologic effect of grafts.
- Grafting of sickle cell ulcers is often unsuccessful.

V EXOGENOUS AGENTS

Introduction

The use of compression is often identified with venous ulcers but we have cared for other types in this way. We commonly use compression bandages with weekly removal by the physician or nurse when we suspect a factitial component to the etiology or persistence of the ulceration. We have also used leg compression successfully as adjunctive therapy in cases of pyoderma gangrenosum and in ulcers developing in fibrotic tissue. However, compression therapy must not be used without first insuring that the leg has good arterial flow. Failure to do so may result in the application of compression to patients with arterial insufficiency, which may lead to tissue necrosis. Therefore we always obtain arterial Doppler studies in limbs that are going to receive compression therapy. An ankle/arm systolic blood pressure under 0.6–0.8 suggests the possibility of significant arterial insufficiency and compression bandages should not be used. We do not know why compression is helpful in some non-venous ulcers but the improvement may be due to better edema removal, greater lymphatic flow, reduced venous pressure and, perhaps, yet uncharacterized effects on cellular and molecular events in the wound.

As we cared for more patients requiring compression therapy, we began to recognize how difficult it is to achieve proper compression. Not only is it virtually impossible for patients to apply their own compression wraps correctly but there is considerable variability in the application by relatively experienced personnel. It should be noted that two schools of thought have evolved in recent years with regard to ulcer compression. Some believe that rigid compression, as with an Unna paste bandage, is ideal because it forces the calf muscle pump up against the hard surface of the boot and increases the efficiency of the pump. Others point out that the Unna boot is unable to adjust to changes in edema and often becomes "loose" for the purpose of compression. They suggest that elastic bandages are better able to adjust to changes in leg volume.

We are not certain who is right but in recent years there has been a convergence of these two main ideas on compression. For example, we now have Unna boots that have a certain "give" or elastic component. A number of clinicians use Unna boots plus elastic wraps. A four-layer bandage is used by others and is said to achieve more consistent compression: it is likely that the use of more than one compression bandage helps by correcting improper application of the first bandage.

In recent years, there has been a virtual explosion in the kinds of occlusive dressings available to clinicians. These dressings achieve moist wound healing and are becoming more accepted by the medical community. Presently, there are four main types: polyurethane films, foams, hydrocolloids and gels. The choice of dressing depends on the clinical situation and whether the clinician wants skin adherence (films and hydrocolloids), transparency (films and gels) or absorbance of exudate (foams, gels and hydrocolloids). We have provided many examples of the use of these dressings. In almost all ulcers, occlusive dressings are able to provide ulcer debridement, pain relief and protection from infection; they can also stimulate granulation tissue development.

16 Compression

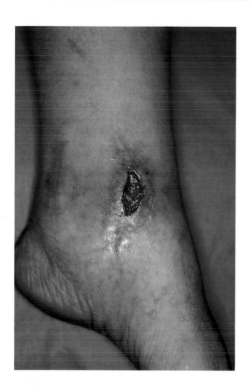

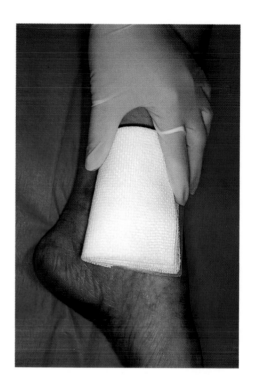

Figure 16.1a
Localized supplemental pressure (LSP)

This young woman developed a persistent ulceration after an injury to her leg. The ulcer persisted in spite of treatment with compression bandages and multiple surgical procedures. Ulcers in this "concave" portion of the leg may not receive adequate pressures during compression treatment. For this reason, we decided to use localized supplemental pressure (LSP), which we have found useful for ulcers in this location.

Figure 16.1b
LSP/Application

Gauze sponges were used directly over the non-healing wound. Other materials may be used.

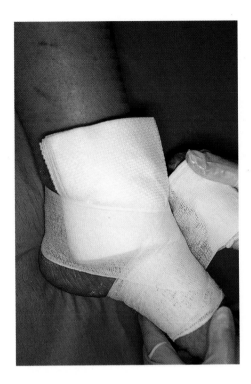

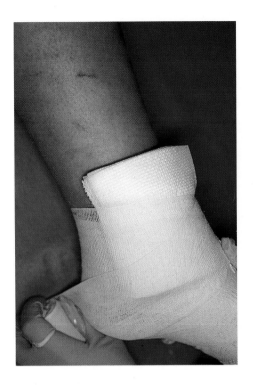

Figure 16.1c
LSP/Application

An Unna paste boot is wrapped around the foot and ankle while maintaining the gauze sponges in place over the ulcer to supplement the pressure of the compression boot.

Figure 16.1d
LSP/Application

As with conventional compression methods, application of the Unna paste boot must include the heel and the mid-portion of the foot.

Continued

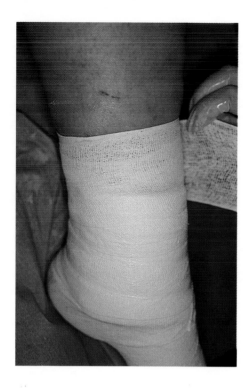

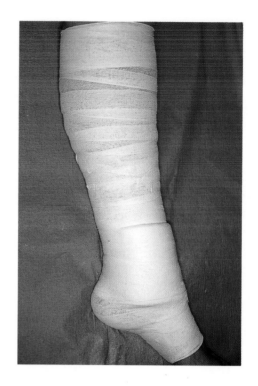

Figure 16.1e
LSP/Application

The wrap is continued over the calf.

Figure 16.1f
LSP/Application

At the end of the application of the Unna boot, the bulge caused by the extra gauze (LSP) is clearly visible.

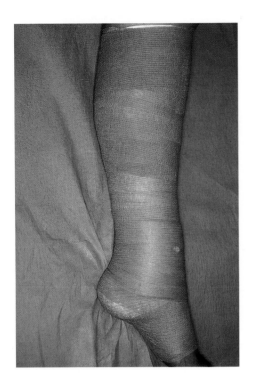

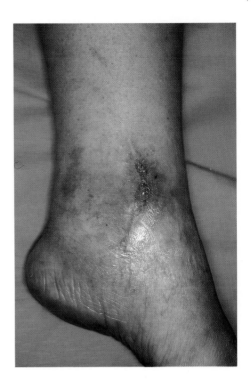

Figure 16.1g
LSP/Application

As in other cases, an extra self-adherent compression wrap was placed over the Unna paste boot to enhance the degree of pressure and keep the underlying bandage in place. The compression and LSP was changed weekly.

Figure 16.1h
LSP/Healing

LSP produced healing in about five weeks.

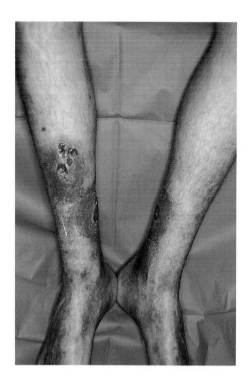

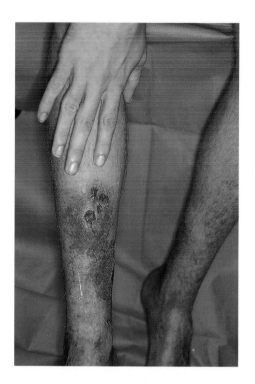

Figure 16.2a
Venous ulcer — rule out homocystinuria

This 21-year-old man had several episodes of severe venous ulcers and venous dermatitis. His mother also has venous ulcers. His hyper-coagulable state is clearly indicated by episodes of pulmonary embolism and thrombosis of his deep iliac system. A hypercoagulable state, early onset of venous disease and venous ulceration, and his body habitus (including long extremities, fingers and toes) led us to consider the diagnosis of homocystinuria. Many attempts have failed to show evidence of homocystinuria. He did not have protein C or S deficiency or the anti-phospholipid syndrome. His ulcers have healed with compression bandages.

Figure 16.2b
Venous ulcer — rule out homocystinuria/ Fingers

The slender fingers with other physical features led us to consider homocystinuria.

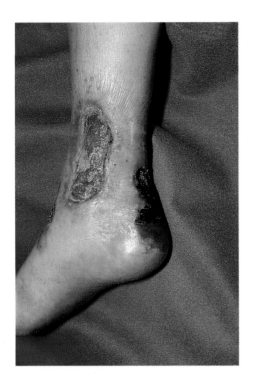

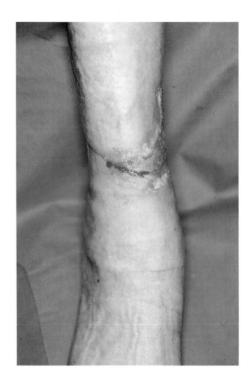

Figure 16.3
Pressure necrosis in arterial disease

The ulcer's location on the medial aspect of the leg and many of its features are consistent with a venous ulcer. The arterial pressure of the leg was not determined before Unna boot therapy was begun. The necrosis over the heel and Achilles tendon is secondary to Unna boot compression in a patient with arterial insufficiency.

Figure 16.4
Immediately after Unna boot removal

The scissors used to cut off the Unna boot lacerated the leg. Blunt scissors and practice preclude this from occurring.

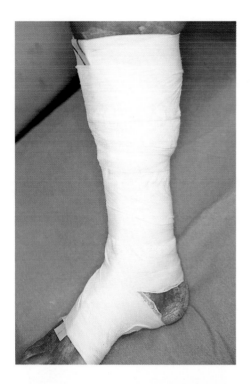

Figure 16.5
Improper compression

This patient's Unna boot was applied incorrectly, leaving the heel unwrapped. Patients often ask us not to wrap their heel.

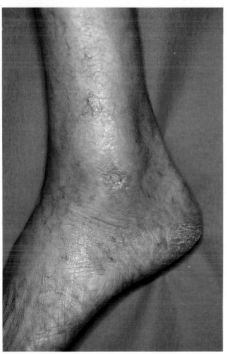

Figure 16.6
Ulcer from small vessel disease

This extremely painful ulcer developed in a patient with a diagnosis of essential thrombocytosis. The ulcer was probably due to the high platelet count and platelet dysfunction observed in that disorder. Although she does not have large vessel arterial disease, compression of the leg should still be avoided in these cases because it may decrease the already compromised blood flow.

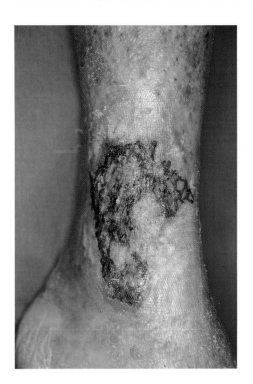

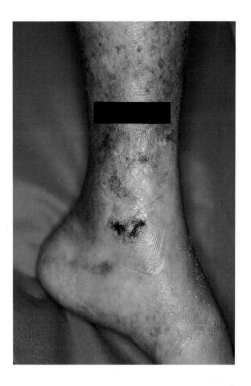

Figure 16.7a
Meshed graft

Two months after split-thickness grafting. We continue Unna boot treatment until, as in this case, there seems to be complete take and graft survival. A self-adherent wrap or, preferably, graded stockings may be applied at this stage.

Figure 16.7b
Meshed graft/Follow up

This shows the same patient about three months later.

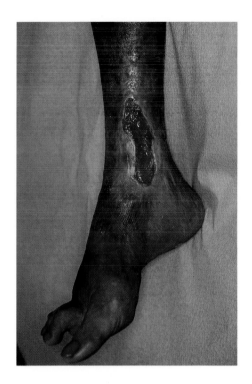

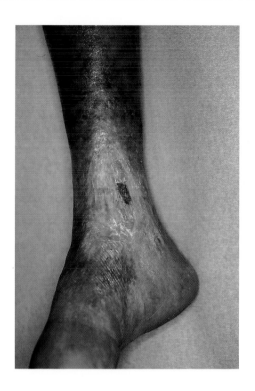

Figure 16.8a
Compression treatment

The venous ulcer in this lady had excellent granulation tissue but had not reepithelialized. She began treatment with elastic compression.

Figure 16.8b
Compression treatment/Follow up

The same patient after three months of treatment.

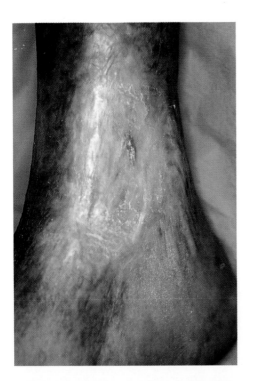

Figure 16.8c
Compression treatment/Follow up

After six months of treatment, the ulcer had just become fully reepithelialized. This sequence of three slides illustrates the often lengthy treatment period needed for full reepithelialization of venous ulcers.

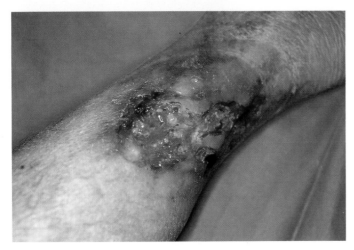

Figure 16.9
Arterial insufficiency

Before using compression therapy one should always exclude arterial disease. This patient had diminished pulses. On Doppler examination and subsequent arteriography he was found to have severe arterial insufficiency. Biopsies did not show cholesterol embolization.

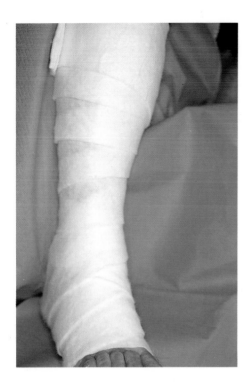

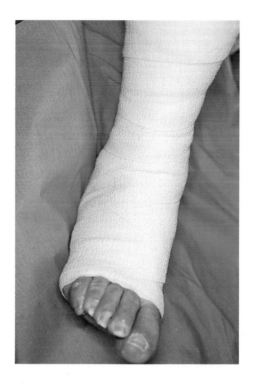

Figure 16.10a
Four-layer bandaging

A novel method of compression has recently been shown to yield better healing rates than conventional bandaging. The method involves the use of four layers of bandages having different properties and elasticity. We suspect that the effectiveness of this method relies on the achievement of more uniform and reliable compression. The first layer, as shown in this photograph, consists of the use of a wool layer, which absorbs exudate and may protect bony prominences from excessive compression.

Figure 16.10b
Four-layer bandaging

The second layer "crepe" bandage adds absorbancy and smooths the underlying wool layer.

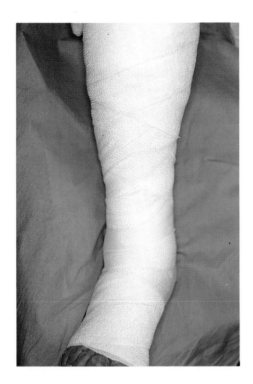 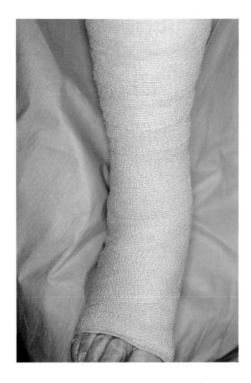

Figure 16.10c
Four-layer bandaging

The third layer, which adds compression, is the only one which is generally applied in a figure of eight. The other layers are applied using the spiral technique of 50% overlap with the preceding turn, as in conventional bandaging.

Figure 16.10d
Four-layer bandaging

The final compression layer is a self-adherent wrap that helps insure proper compression.

17 Dressings

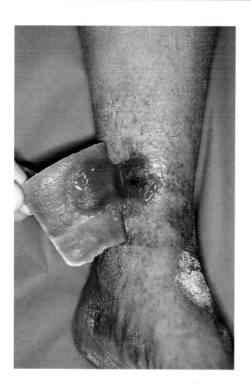

Figure 17.1
Removing a hydrocolloid dressing

The brown-yellow material that accumulates under the dressing is frequently mistaken for pus.

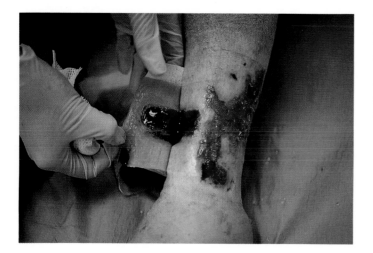

Figure 17.2
Bloody exudate beneath an occlusive dressing

A bloody exudate is not common, and it appears to have no special significance.

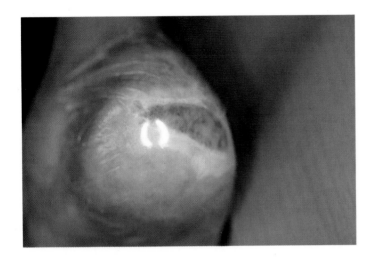

Figure 17.3a
Polyurethane film dressing

A film was used to stimulate granulation tissue formation in this neuropathic heel ulcer. After a few days, fluid had accumulated beneath the dressing. This is expected and patients treated with occlusive dressings are told not to change the dressing until it leaks.

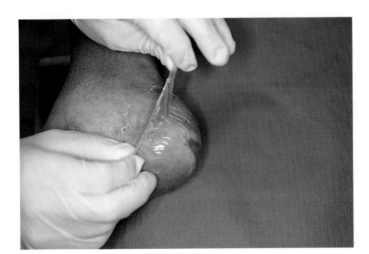

Figure 17.3b
Polyurethane film dressing/ Removal

It is often tempting to remove films by rolling them back. We advise against this method which, evidence shows, causes greater force per unit area than simply lifting the dressing as a sheet (see next two illustrations).

Continued

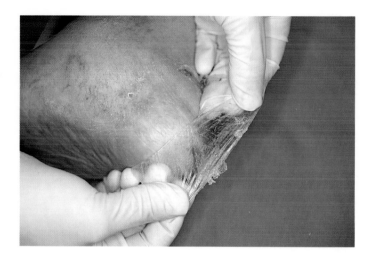

Figure 17.3c
**Polyurethane film dressing/
Removal**

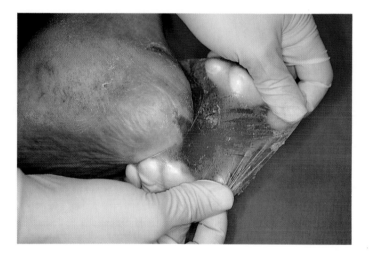

Figure 17.3d
**Polyurethane film dressing/
Removal**

After complete removal of the
dressing the ulcer is irrigated gently
and a new film is applied.

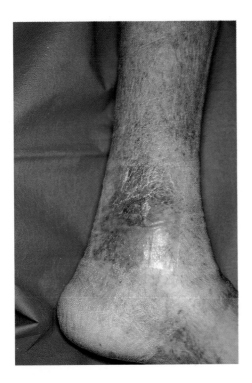

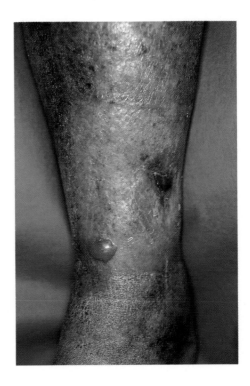

Figure 17.4
Ulcer due to cryoglobulinemia

The intractable pain caused by this ulcer was promptly relieved by a polyurethane film occlusive dressing. Initially, the ulcer was necrotic but several days of occlusive dressing treatment has not only relieved the pain but induced a painless debridement. Pain relief and painless debridement are major benefits of occlusive dressing therapy.

Figure 17.5
Blister beneath an occlusive dressing

We have only seen this in two patients. The blister does not appear to be the result of removing the hydrocolloid dressing but it is seen upon removal. Occlusive dressing therapy was discontinued. However, we cannot be certain that the blister was caused by the dressing.

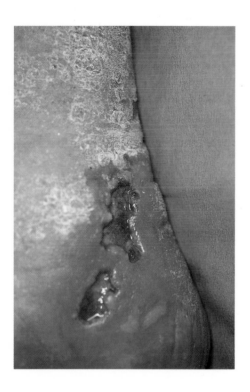

Figure 17.6
Blister under an occlusive dressing

This patient with sickle cell disease had very painful ulcers near the Achilles tendon. A gel dressing relieved the pain dramatically. When the dressing was removed a blister was seen (lower portion of this field). We have noted these blisters in some patients treated with occlusive dressings; but we do not know whether the blistering is caused by the dressing.

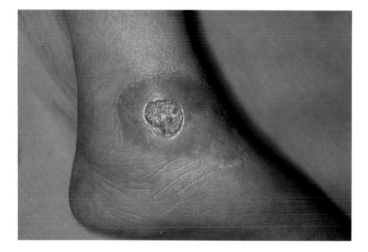

Figure 17.7
Venous ulcer in a patient with multiple sclerosis

This middle aged lady virtually lives in her wheel chair. The redness and edema around the ulcer is secondary to an occlusive dressing.

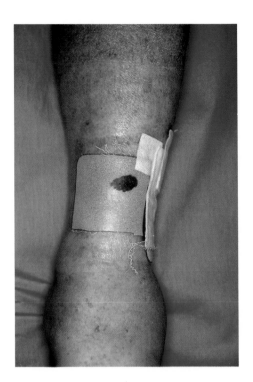

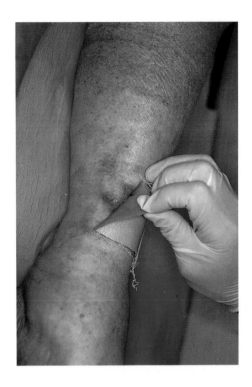

Figure 17.8a
Removal of a hydrocolloid dressing

A hydrocolloid dressing was used to relieve pain, stimulate granulation tissue and cause painless debridement in this patient with cryoglobuline-mia. Before removal, an area of bloody exudate is apparent on the surface of the dressing. Removal is not necessitated by this appearance so long as there is no "breakthrough" or leaking of the exudate. We encourage patients to leave these dressings on as long as possible and in some cases patients have a "wearing time" of 10 to 12 days.

Figure 17.8b
Removal of a hydrocolloid dressing

This and the following four photographs illustrate removal of the hydrocolloid. This is done gently and carefully to minimize injury from the adherent dressing to the underlying intact epidermis. During this procedure, we often stop and irrigate the area to facilitate removal.

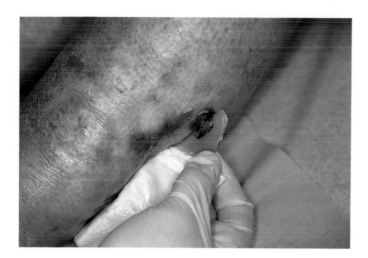

Figure 17.8c
Removal of a hydrocolloid dressing

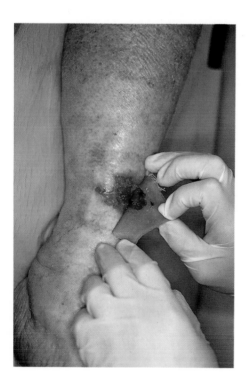

Figure 17.8d
Removal of a hydrocolloid dressing

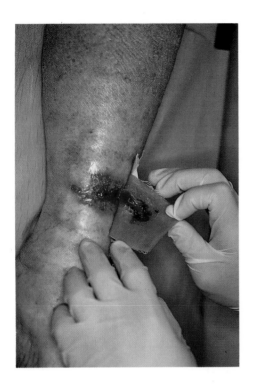

Figure 17.8e
Removal of a hydrocolloid dressing

The dressing does not adhere to the wound itself, but rather it "melts" into the wound. The brown/yellow exudate that is often observed with the use of occlusive dressings is the result of wound fluid plus hydrocolloid dressing material.

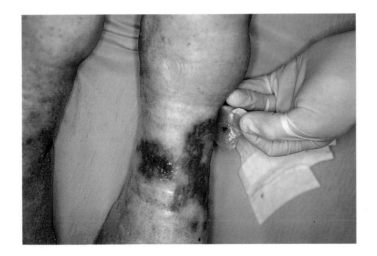

Figure 17.8f
Removal of a hydrocolloid dressing

A new dressing is generally applied after gentle irrigation of the wound.

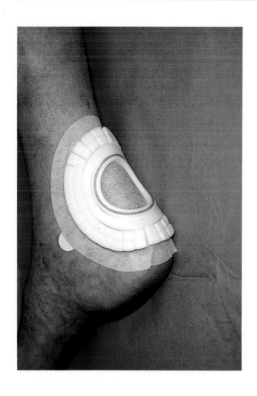

Figure 17.9
Pressure relief

This type of dressing, a hydrocolloid with removable foam rings, is mainly used in decubitus (pressure) ulcers. We have found it helpful in patients with pressure ulcers of the lower extremity.

Clinical points

- Certain parts of ulcers may not receive adequate compression. One can remedy this by applying additional bandages between the ulcer and compression wraps (localized supplemental pressure).

- Arterial insufficiency should be excluded before the application of compression wraps.

- Compression wraps, including Unna boots, must always be applied so as to include the heel.

- Compression therapy seems to help the "take" of split-thickness skin grafts.

- The yellow/brown, and often malodorous, material that accumulates under some hydrocolloid dressings is frequently mistaken for pus. Patients need to be warned.

- Occlusive dressings should not be removed until the fluid that has accumulated under the dressing causes it to leak.

- Occlusive dressings reduce the pain of most ulcers, even those due to cryoglobulinemia.

Glossary of selected terms

Air plethysmography

A reliable and reproducible way to assess venous disease. The method takes advantage of volume measurements of the calf after inflation of a cuff around it. It can give values for volume and ejection fraction.

Antiphospholipid syndrome

A constellation of clinical features due to a hypercoagulable state occurring in an idiopathic form or in association with collagen vascular diseases, particularly systemic lupus erythematosus. The syndrome is due to the presence of antibodies directed against phospholipids. Diagnosis is aided by finding a false positive VDRL, anticardiolipin antibodies, and an elevated partial thromboplastin time that is not correctable by the addition of normal plasma (lupus anticoagulant).

Arterial Doppler studies

These are useful in screening patients for the presence of arterial insufficiency. For lower extremity measurements, the sensor is placed over either the dorsalis pedis or posterior tibialis pulse. The ratio of the ankle systolic pressure to the brachial arterial pressure (normally slightly greater than 1.0) is called the ankle brachial index (ABI). Patients with an ABI less than 0.7 should be investigated further for the presence of significant arterial insufficiency.

Atrophie blanche

A poorly understood clinical entity manifested by avascular or poorly vascularized skin areas often studded with dot-like capillaries. It is not a clearly defined clinical diagnosis and is seen in many vascular conditions, including venous and arterial disease, vasculitis, cryoglobulinemia and cryofibrinogenemia, and collagen vascular diseases. In several of these conditions intravascular fibrin thrombi can be detected histologically.

Cholesterol embolization

Cholesterol crystals separating from larger atheromatous plaques and embolizing to small vessels in the skin and other organs can give rise to a distinctive syndrome which includes but is not restricted to the following features: constitutional symptoms, sudden hypertension, renal failure, CNS disturbances, livedo reticularis and skin ulceration.

Clofazimine

A drug used to treat leprosy. It has been reported to be useful in the treatment of pyoderma gangrenosum.

Cryofibrinogenemia

The presence in plasma of fibrinogen that is precipitable by cold temperature. It can occur in an idiopathic form or associated with collagen vascular diseases, vascular thrombosis, and malignancy. Cryofibrinogen is in plasma, whereas cryoglobulins are detected in serum. Symptomatic patients may suffer from vascular thrombosis, livedo reticularis, purpura and skin ulceration. The cutaneous manifestations may respond dramatically to treatment with stanozolol.

Cryoglobulinemia

The presence in blood of proteins that are precipitable by cold temperature. It may be idiopathic, but is often associated with collagen vascular diseases, vasculitis, and malignancy, particularly lymphomas and leukemias.

Eosinophilic fasciitis

This starts typically with swelling of the hands and/or feet. The tense edema gives rise to a characteristic peau d'orange appearance of the skin. The edematous phase is quickly followed by progressive joint contractures and induration of the extremities which spares the digits.

Lipodermatosclerosis (LDS)

This refers to the induration that develops most often on the medial aspect of the leg in patients with venous disease. Clinically and histologically, LDS is probably the same condition as dermatitis sclerodermiformis and sclerosing panniculitis. There is an acute phase, manifested by pain, tenderness, erythema, scaling and induration, which is followed by the chronic phase of hyperpigmentation and painless induration. Acute LDS may respond dramatically to treatment with stanozolol.

Livedo reticularis

This is a net-like reticulated non-blanchable pattern of erythema and hyperpigmentation that is related to skin vascular damage. It is most common on the lower extremities but may also involve the trunk, as observed with cholesterol embolization. Livedo reticularis is also associated with vasculitis, antiphospholipid syndrome and cryoproteinemias.

Necrobiosis lipoidica diabeticorum

Atrophic, yellow to red discoloration of the skin usually over the shin. It is pathognomonic for diabetes mellitus: patients either have diabetes, or will develop diabetes, or have a strong family history of diabetes. It occasionally ulcerates.

Occlusive dressings (OD)

A class of agents that allow moist wound healing. OD enhance reepithelialization of acute wounds and have been shown to relieve pain and stimulate granulation tissue in chronic wounds. Increasing evidence suggests that their use is associated with decreased scarring. There are five main types of OD depending on their composition, oxygen and water vapor permeability, and adhesiveness: films, hydrocolloids, foams, alginates, and gels.

Pericapillary fibrin (PCF)

The presence of fibrin deposits in and around capillaries. PCF is detectable by direct immunofluorescence in virtually all cases of venous disease, where it is not associated with other immunoreactants. It is composed mostly of undegraded fibrin. PCF is helpful in confirming the diagnosis of lipodermatosclerosis in uncertain clinical cases but is not specific for venous disease.

Photoplethysmography

A non-invasive test for the presence of venous insufficiency. An infrared sensor is placed over a suitable area of the lower extremity, usually the medial aspect of the ankle. Rapid emptying of the venous blood from the lower extremity by repeated dorsiflexion or other suitable excercise, allows the sensor to detect the venous refilling time.

Pulse intravenous steroid therapy

The intravenous administration of pharmacologic doses of corticosteroids over a finite period of time. This use of corticosteroids appears to be associated with fewer long term side effects. Typically, 1 g of methylprednisolone is given intravenously over several minutes every day for three to five days. Careful monitoring of electrolytes is necessary and, in patients on diuretics, telemetry should be used.

Pyoderma gangrenosum (PG)

A rapidly enlarging ulceration that is typified by purple edges, undermined borders and by net-like epidermal resurfacing (cribriform pattern). The amount of subcutaneous necrosis can be extensive, but the ulcer bed looks generally clean without evidence of infection. PG is commonly idiopathic but is also associated with rheumatoid arthritis, other collagen vascular diseases, ulcerative colitis, leukemia, Behçet's disease, and idiopathic IgA gammopathy.

Retinoic acid

A derivative of vitamin A that is normally used to treat acne vulgaris. As with its parent compound, it has profound effects on cellular differentiation. When applied topically to a poorly granulating wound bed in immunocompromised patients, retinoic acid may restore and accelerate the formation of granulation tissue.

Stanozolol

An anabolic steroid with attenuated androgenic effects. Stanozolol has fibrinolytic activity but the mode of action is not fully understood. It leads to remarkable improvement in the tenderness and induration associated with lipodermatosclerosis, and has been found to cause dramatic pain relief and ulcer healing in patients with ulcers due to cryofibrinogenemia. Doses as low as 2 mg twice a day result in therapeutic effects. Stanozolol causes sodium retention and should not be used in patients with uncontrolled hypertension or a history of congestive heart failure. Other notable side effects include elevation of liver function tests, decreased HDL and hirsutism.

Venous hypertension

In normal standing individuals, venous pressure in the legs is the hydrostatic pressure measured from the level of the heart to the feet. Upon walking or leg exercise, the venous pressure in the lower extremities decreases. This is due to the action of the calf-muscle pump which drives blood from the superficial veins into the deep venous system and back to the heart. In patients with a damaged venous system or faulty calf-muscle pump action the expected fall of the venous pressure with ambulation or exercise does not occur. This situation is termed venous hypertension. Venous hypertension is the underlying cause of venous ulceration, although the pathogenic steps involved are not understood.

Wood's light

A light (black light) that emits ultraviolet A. It is particularly helpful in detecting a heavy burden of *Pseudomonas aeruginosa* in ulcerated tissue. This is because Pseudomonas secretes a substance that fluoresces green with ultraviolet A radiation.

Zinc chloride paste

A preparation that was originally developed for tissue fixation prior to Mohs surgery for microscopically controlled removal of skin cancer. The zinc chloride fixes the tissue, hardens it, and makes it slough or easier to remove. It has been used for tissue debridement.

Selected bibliography

Bays HE, Pfeifer MA
Peripheral diabetic neuropathy. *Med Clin North Am* (1988) **72**:1439–1464.

Bizer LS, Ramos S, Weiss PR
A prospective randomized double blind study of perioperative antibiotic use in the grafting of ulcers of the lower extremity. *Surg Gynecol Obstet* (1992) **175**:113–114.

Black MM, Walkden VM
Basal cell carcinomatous changes on the lower leg: a possible association with chronic venous stasis. *Histopathology* (1983) **7**:219–227.

Blauvelt A, Falanga V
Idiopathic and L-tryptophan associated eosinophilic fasciitis before and after L-tryptophan contamination. *Arch Dermatol* (1991) **127**:1159–1166.

Boulton AJM
The diabetic foot. *Med Clin North Am* (1988) **72**:1513–1529.

Brodland DG, Staats BA, Peters MS
Factitial leg ulcers associated with an unusual sleep disorder. *Arch Dermatol* (1989) **125**:1115–1118.

Browse NL, Burnand KG
The cause of venous ulceration. *Lancet* (1982) **ii**:243–245.

Browse NL, Gray L, Jarrett PEM, et al
Blood and vein-wall fibrinolytic activity in health and vascular disease. *Br Med J* (1977) **275**:478-481.

Burnand K, Clemenson G, Morland M, et al
Venous lipodermatosclerosis: treatment by fibrinolytic enhancement and elastic compression. *Br Med J* (1980) **280**:7–11.

Burnand K, Lea Thomas M, O'Donnell T, et al
Relation between postphlebitic changes in the deep veins and results of surgical treatment of venous ulcers. *Lancet* (1976) **i**:936–938.

Callam MJ, Harper DR, Dale JJ, et al
Chronic ulcer of the leg: clinical history. *Br Med J* (1987) **294**:1389–1391.

Callam MJ, Harper DR, Dale JJ, et al
A controlled trial of weekly ultrasound therapy in chronic leg ulceration. *Lancet* (1987) **ii**:204–206.

Clark RAF
Basis of cutaneous wound repair. *J Dermatol Surg Oncol* (1993) **19**:693–706.

Claudy AL, Mirshahi M, Soria C, et al
Detection of undegraded fibrin and tumor necrosis factor-alpha in venous leg ulcers. *J Am Acad Dermatol* (1991) **25**:623–627.

Coleridge Smith P, Sarin Sanjeev, Hasty J, et al
Sequential gradient pneumatic compression enhances venous ulcer healing: a randomized trial. *Surgery* (1990) **108**:871–875.

Colgan M-P, Dormandy JA, Jones PW, et al
Oxpentifylline treatment of venous ulcers of the leg. *Br Med J* (1990) **300**:972–975.

De Ceulaer K, Khamashta MA, Harris EN, et al
Antiphospholipid antibodies in homozygous sickle cell disease. *Ann Rheum Dis* (1992) **51**:671–672.

Don Park S, Sun Shon H, Joong Joh N
Vibrio vulnificus septicemia in Korea: clinical and epidemiologic findings in seventy patients. *J Am Acad Dermatol* (1991) **24**:397–403.

Dvorak HF
Tumors: wounds that do not heal. *N Engl J Med* (1986) **315**:1650–1659.

Eaglstein WH, Davis SC, Mehle AI, et al
Optimal use of an occlusive dressing to enhance healing: effect of delayed application and early removal on wound healing. *Arch Dermatol* (1988) **124**:392–395.

Elgart G, Stover P, Larson K, et al
Treatment of pyoderma gangrenosum with cyclosporine: results in seven patients. *J Am Acad Dermatol* (1991) **24**:83–86.

English MP, Smith RJ, Harman RRM
The fungal flora of ulcerated legs. *Br J Dermatol* (1971) **84**:567–582.

Falanga V
Occlusive wound dressings: why, when, which? *Arch Dermatol* (1988) **124**:872–877.

Falanga V
Chronic wounds: pathophysiologic and experimental considerations. *J Invest Dermatol* (1993) **100**:721–725.

Falanga V, Eaglstein WH
A therapeutic approach to venous ulcers. *J Am Acad Dermatol* (1986) **14**:777–784.

Falanga V, Eaglstein WH
The trap hypothesis of venous ulceration. *Lancet* (1993) **341**:1006–1008.

Falanga V, Iriondo M
Zinc chloride paste for the debridement of chronic leg ulcers. *J Dermatol Surg Oncol* (1990) **16**:658–661.

Falanga V, Kirsner RS, Eaglstein WH, et al
Stanozolol in treatment of leg ulcers due to cryofibrinogenemia. *Lancet* (1991) **338**:347–348.

Falanga V, Kirsner RS, Katz MH, et al
Pericapillary fibrin cuffs in venous ulceration. *J Dermatol Surg Oncol* (1992) **18**:409–414.

Falanga V, Kruskal JB, Franks JJ
Fibrin and fibrinogen-related antigens in patients with venous disease and venous ulceration. *Arch Dermatol* (1991) **127**:75–78.

Falanga V, McKenzie A, Eaglstein WH
Heterogeneity in oxygen diffusion around venous ulcers. *J Dermatol Surg Oncol* (1991) **13**:336–339.

Falanga V, Moosa HH, Nemeth AJ, et al
Dermal pericapillary fibrin in venous ulceration. *Arch Dermatol* (1987) **123**:620–623.

Falstie-Jensen N, Spaun E, Brochner-Mortensen J, et al
The influence of epidermal thickness on transcutaneous oxygen pressure measurements in normal persons. *Scand J Clin Lab Invest* (1988) **48**:519–523.

Fine MJ, Kapoor W, Falanga V
Cholesterol crystal embolization: a review of 221 cases in the English literature. *Angiology* (1987) **38**:769–784.

Fraki JE, Peltonen L, Hopsu-Havu VK
Allergy to various components of topical preparations in stasis dermatitis and leg ulcer. *Contact Dermatitis* (1979) **5**:97–100.

Gilchrist B, Reed C
The bacteriology of chronic venous ulcers treated with occlusive hydrocolloid dressings. *Br J Dermatol* (1989) **121**:337–344.

Gilman TH
Parameter for measurement of wound closure. *Wounds* (1990) **3**:95–101.

Gowland Hopkins NF, Jamieson CW
Antibiotic concentration in the exudate of venous ulcers: the prediction of healing rate. *Br J Surg* (1983) **70**:532–534.

Gowland Hopkins NF, Spinks TJ, Rhodes CG, et al
Positron emission tomography in venous ulceration and liposclerosis: study of regional tissue function. *Br Med J* (1983) **286**:333–336.

Grob JJ, San Marco M, Aillaud MF, et al
Unfading acral microlivedo. A discrete marker of thrombotic skin disease associated with antiphospholipid antibody syndrome. *J Am Acad Dermatol* (1991) **24**:53–58.

Harris B, Eaglstein WH, Falanga V
Basal cell carcinoma arising in venous ulcers and mimicking granulation tissue. *J Dermatol Surg Oncol* (1993) **19**:150–152.

Harrison PV
Split-skin grafting of varicose leg ulcers — a survey and the importance of assessment of risk factors in predicting outcome from the procedure. *Clin Exp Dermatol* (1988) **13**:4–6.

Hendricks WM, Swallow RT
Management of stasis leg ulcers with Unna's boots versus elastic support stockings. *J Am Acad Dermatol* (1985) **12**:90–98.

Hook EW, Hooton TM, Horton CA, et al
Microbiologic evaluation of cutaneous cellulitis in adults. *Arch Intern Med* (1986) **146**:295–297.

Hunt TK, Ehrlich HP, Garcia JA, et al
Effect of vitamin A on reversing the inhibitory effect of cortisone on healing of open wounds in animals and man. *Ann Surg* (1969) **170**:633–641.

Johnson G, Kupper C, Farrar DJ, et al
Graded compression stockings. Custom vs noncustom. *Arch Surg* (1982) **117**:69–72.

Johnson RB, Lazarus GS
Pulse therapy. Therapeutic efficacy in the treatment of pyoderma gangrenosum. *Arch Dermatol* (1982) **118**:76–84.

Katz MH, Alvarez AF, Kirsner RS, et al
Human wound fluid from acute wounds stimulates fibroblast and endothelial cell growth. *J Am Acad Dermatol* (1991) **25**:1054–1058.

Kirsner RS, Falanga V, Eaglstein WH
The biology of skin grafts: skin grafts as pharmacologic agents. *Arch Dermatol* (1993) **129**:481–483.

Kirsner RS, Pardes JB, Eaglstein WH, et al
The clinical spectrum of lipodermatosclerosis. *J Am Acad Dermatol* (1993) **28**:623–627.

Klein KL, Pittelkow MR
Tissue plasminogen activator for treatment of livedoid vasculitis. *Mayo Clin Proc* (1992) **67**:923–933.

Lewis CE, Antoine J, Mueller C, et al
Elastic compression in the prevention of venous stasis. A critical reevaluation. *Am J Surg* (1976) **132**:739–743.

LoGerfo FW, Coffman JD
Vascular and microvascular disease of the foot in diabetes. *N Engl J Med* (1984) **311**:1615–1619.

Lookingbill DP, Miller SH, Knowles RC
Bacteriology of chronic leg ulcers. *Arch Dermatol* (1978) **114**:1765–1768.

Mitchell Sams W
Livedo vasculitis. Therapy with pentoxifylline. *Arch Dermatol* (1988) **124**:684–687.

Moosa HH, Falanga V, Steed DL, et al
Oxygen diffusion in chronic venous ulceration. *J Cardiovasc Surg* (1987) **28**:464–467.

Myers MB, Rightor M, Cherry GW
Relationship between edema and the healing rate of stasis ulcers of the leg. *Am J Surg* (1972) **124**:66–68.

Nemeth AJ, Eaglstein WH, Falanga V
Clinical parameters and transcutaneous oxygen measurements for the prognosis of venous ulcers. *J Am Acad Dermatol* (1989) **20**:186–190.

Newman LG, Waller J, Palestro CJ, et al
Unsuspected osteomyelitis in diabetic foot ulcers. *JAMA* (1991) **266**:1246–1251.

Partsch H
Compression therapy of the legs. A review. *J Dermatol Surg Oncol* (1991) **17**:799–805.

Pathy AL, Rae V, Falanga V
Subcutaneous calcification in venous ulcers. *J Dermatol Surg Oncol* (1990) **16**:450–452.

Phillips TJ, Kehinde O, Green H, et al
Treatment of skin ulcers with cultured epidermal allografts. *J Am Acad Dermatol* (1989) **21**:191–199.

Phillips TJ, Salman SM, Rogers GS
Nonhealing leg ulcers: a manifestation of basal cell carcinoma. *J Am Acad Dermatol* (1991) **25**:47–49.

Prasad A, Ali-Khan A, Mortimer PS
Leg ulcers and oedema: a study exploring the prevalence, aetiology, and possible significance of oedema in venous ulcers. *Phlebology* (1990) **5**:181–187.

Rademaker M, Lowe DG, Munro DD
Erythema induratum (Bazin's disease). *J Am Acad Dermatol* (1989) **21**:740–745.

Rae V, Pardo RJ, Blackwelder PL, et al
Leg ulcers following large volume subcutaneous injection of liquid silicone preparation. *Arch Dermatol* (1989) **125**:670–673.

Ram Zvi, Sadeh M, Walden R, et al
Vascular insufficiency quantitatively aggravates diabetic neuropathy. *Arch Neurol* (1991) **48**:1239–1242.

Sarin S, Cheatle TR, Coleridge Smith PD, et al
Disease mechanisms in venous ulceration. *Br J Hosp Med* (1991) **45**:303–305.

Scheffler A, Rieger H
A comparative analysis of transcutaneous oxymetry (tcPO$_2$) during oxygen inhalation and leg dependency in severe peripheral arterial occlusive disease. *J Vasc Surg* (1992) **16**:218–224.

Serjeant GR
Leg ulceration in sickle cell anemia. *Arch Intern Med* (1974) **133**:690–694.

Sigel B, Edelstein AL, Savitch L, et al
Type of compression for reducing venous stasis. A study of lower extremities during inactive recumbency. *Arch Surg* (1975) **110**:171–175.

Sindrup JH, Groth S, Avnstorp C, et al
Coexistence of obstructive arterial disease and chronic venous stasis in leg ulcer patients. *Clin Exp Dermatol* (1987) **12**:410–412.

Skene AI, Smith JM, Dore CJ, et al
Venous leg ulcers: a prognostic index to predict time to healing. *Br Med J* (1992) **305**:1119–1121.

Smith RJ, English MP, Warin RP
The pathogenic status of yeasts infecting ulcerated legs. *Br J Dermatol* (1974) **91**:697–699.

Stacey MC, Burnand KG, Layer GT, et al
Transcutaneous oxygen tensions in assessing the treatment of healed venous ulcers. *Br J Surg* (1990) **77**:1050–1054.

Vanscheidt W, Laaff H, Weiss JM, et al
Immunohistochemical investigation of dermal capillaries in chronic venous insufficiency. *Acta Derm Venereol (Stockh)* (1991) **71**:17–19.

Wieman JT, Griffiths GD, Polk HC
Management of diabetic midfoot ulcers. *Ann Surg* (1992) **215**:627–632.

Woods GL, Washington JA
Mycobacteria other than Mycobacterium tuberculosis: review of microbiologic and clinical aspects. *Rev Infect Dis* (1987) **9**:275–294.

Yao ST, Hobbs JT, Irvine WT
Ankle systolic pressure measurements in arterial disease affecting the lower extremities. *Br J Surg* (1969) **56**:676–679.

Index